W9-AYX-921

ONE MEAL
A DAY DIET

Lose 1 Pound a Day and Lose 10 Pounds in a Week with Intermittent Fasting

DIANA POLSKA

Copyright © 2017 by Diana Polska

All rights reserved. No part of this book may be reproduced or transmitted in any form or by any electronic or mechanical means, including photo-copy, recording, or any information storage and retrieval system now known or to be invented, without written permission from the author, except by a reviewer who wishes to quote brief passages in connection with a review written for inclusion in a magazine, newspaper, website, or broadcast.

Disclaimer: Neither the author nor the publisher shall be held liable or responsible to any person or entity with respect to any loss or incidental or consequential damages caused, directly or indirectly, by the information or programs contained herein. You must seek the services of a competent professional before beginning any health or weight-loss advice. References are provided for informational purposes only. They do not constitute endorsement of any websites or other sources.

DEDICATION

This book is dedicated to all who have tried unsuccessfully to lose weight and who feel like it may never be possible. It's for those who not only want to look good, but also feel good, improve their health, and have higher energy levels.

CONTENTS

PREFACE

When he was younger, a man conducted an experiment. He was raising a pig for the state fair. He fed his pig at a specific time of the day, allowing the pig to eat as much as it wanted but only at a specific time, following a feeding schedule based on meal frequency and meal timing.

His friends fed their pigs the traditional way, letting the pigs have access to food all day and allowing them to eat whenever they wanted (at all times during the day).

When it came time for judging, the man's pig had grown to be very strong, healthy, and LEAN, while his friends' pigs had grown fat.

Pigs are not known for their lean figures; therefore, the man who had raised the lean pig, who himself was overweight, was convinced that he had found the secret to losing weight and keeping it off. He decided to use the exact method in which he fed his lean state fair pig. He ate as much as he wanted and ate whatever he wanted, but he ate at specific times during the day. He lost 42 pounds in two years and has kept it off for seven years and counting.

The man's very successful experiment is in line with the groundbreaking weight loss research conducted recently on meal timing and frequency.

This book contains over 700 scientific references. It is a collection of all the latest research and the growing body of scientific evidence to support the health and weight-loss benefits of meal frequency, meal timing, and intermittent fasting.

The One Meal a Day Diet, also called the OMAD Diet, is a method of losing weight that is based on intermittent fasting, meal frequency, and meal timing. It's an easy and fast way to get thin and stay thin forever (no more yo-yo weight battles). It's possible to eat whatever you want and still lose weight.

The OMAD Diet is not a temporary weight-loss method or fad diet. It's a lifestyle plan that works for the long-term. This scientifically-based, comprehensive lifestyle plan works simply because, unlike short-term weight-loss diets, an easy-to-follow, lifelong weight-management lifestyle will help you lose weight and keep it off permanently. In addition, it will dramatically improve your health, energy, and well-being.

I wrote this book because I'm so tired of seeing people go on temporary diets and lose weight, then regain the weight—and in many cases gain back even more than they lost.

The information in this book is based on recent groundbreaking scientific studies. We will also examine the lifestyles and eating habits that allow certain nationalities, like the French, to eat fatty foods and desserts while remaining thin.

Going on short-term weight-loss diets is very unhealthy and leads to increased weight gain over time. Weight cycling is the repeated loss and regain of body weight. Studies show that weight cycling is linked to an increased waist-to-hip ratio (WHR).[1] A stable weight maintained over time is associated with the best health status.[2]

We already know that a proper, balanced diet is one of the essential keys to an ideal weight, good health, and the prevention of diseases such as cardiovascular disease, cancer, diabetes, Alzheimer's disease, cataracts, dental disease, and osteoporosis.[3] The problem is that an overwhelming amount of information exists about what constitutes a healthy diet. For any person who reads a lot or listens to health gurus and experts, knowing how to eat well can be confusing. There are all sort of diets: vegetarian, low-fat, raw, alkaline, vegan, blood-type, high-protein, low-carb, ketogenic, macrobiotic, Mediterranean, Paleo, and gluten-free, to name just a few.

The beauty of The OMAD Diet is that you don't have to starve yourself or count calories. It's a simple method: You eat only once per day and do high-intensity interval training (HIIT).

There are two strategies to the OMAD diet. You can eat once per day, do HIIT, and eat any types of food that you want. However, if you want to speed up your weight loss results, the other option is to eat the types of foods recommended in Chapter 2. It really depends on how fast you want to lose weight and whether you need to improve your health. You can skip Chapter 2 if you don't want to eat specific foods and don't have any major health concerns.

INTRODUCTION

The World Health Organization (WHO) defines obesity as abnormal or excessive fat accumulation that presents a risk to health. Obesity is a health concern, as it is a risk factor for many common chronic diseases such as heart disease and stroke, diabetes mellitus, osteoarthritis, and hypertension. The WHO estimates that being overweight or obese leads directly to the death of at least 2.8 million adults every year worldwide.

Current guidelines use the body mass index (BMI) to define obesity. All adults aged 20 years and older are evaluated on the same BMI scale as follows:

- Underweight: BMI below 18.5
- Normal weight: BMI 18.5 to 24.9
- Overweight: BMI 25.0 to 29.9
- Obese: BMI 30 and above

In addition to calculating your BMI, measuring body fat percentage is a good way to determine weight status. BMI factors in only your height and weight. It will give you the same reading if you have 160 pounds of pure muscle or 160 pounds of pure fat. Body fat percentage is the percentage of weight that is pure fat.

The tendency toward a body type with an unusually high number of fat cells—termed endomorphic—appears to be inherited. Other genetic factors influence appetite and the metabolic rate at which food is transformed into energy. Although inheritance may play a role, a genetic predisposition toward weight gain does not in itself cause obesity. Family eating habits are major contributors to the development of obesity.

Occasionally, obesity does have a purely physiological cause:

- Cushing's syndrome, a disorder involving the excessive release of the hormone cortisol

- Hypothyroidism, caused by an under-active thyroid gland, resulting in low levels of the hormone thyroxin and the slow metabolism of food and calories stored as fat

- Some cases of hypoglycemia, or low blood sugar, due to a metabolic disorder that results in carbohydrates being stored as fat

- Neurological disturbances, such as damage to the hypothalamus, a structure located deep within the brain that helps regulate appetite

- Certain drugs, such as steroids, antipsychotic medications, and antidepressants

Check with a medical doctor or naturopathic doctor to rule out any purely physiological causes of weight gain.

The WHO states that "the fundamental cause of obesity and overweight is an energy imbalance between calories consumed and calories expended." However, lowering calorie intake and increasing energy expenditure is easier said than done, and most weight-loss programs are experimental and lack validation through scientific research.[1][2]

Diets to promote weight loss are generally divided into four categories: low-fat, low-carbohydrate, low-calorie, and very low calorie. Research has found that none of these common weight-loss diets helps a person lose weight in the long run.[3]

Long-term studies indicate that the majority of people who lose weight by dieting end up regaining all the weight they lost regardless of whether they maintained their diet or exercise programs.[4] After two years of dieting, up to two-thirds of dieters are even heavier than they were prior to beginning their regimens. Therefore, the American Psychological Association has concluded that diets do not lead to sustained weight loss or health benefits for the majority of people.

Some claim that there is no point in losing weight because it's genetic or some simply come to understand that diets don't work. While there are some rare genetic conditions that cause obesity, and while most diets don't work, there is no reason why most people cannot lose weight with the proper knowledge. A genetic predisposition toward weight gain does not in itself cause obesity.[5][6] "Knowledge is power," said Francis Bacon. Determining the root cause of weight gain will help you solve the problem for good.

WHY OBESITY HAS SOARED

America is number one on the 2013 top 10 list of countries with the most obese citizens. In America, it is a common habit to eat three meals plus two to five snacks every day. According to the National Health and Nutrition Examination Survey 1999-2000, 80 percent of all Americans eat at least four or five times per day.

The frequency of eating due to snacking has increased over the past 30 years in the U.S.[7] As snacking frequency has increased throughout the years, so have the rates of obesity. From 1950 through 1960, 9.7 percent of U.S. adults were obese. In 2012, more than one-third (34.9 percent) of U.S. adults—a total of 78.6 million—were obese.[8]

Besides meal frequency, the method of food preparation has changed and this has contributed to the rise in obesity rates. In the 1960s, families cooked their own food and ate it at home. Since then, technological innovations—including vacuum packing, improved preservatives, artificial flavors, and microwaves—have made food more available for rapid consumption.

In 1965, a married woman spent over two hours per day cooking and cleaning up from meals. In 1995, the same tasks took less than half that time.

Food is now fast to prepare and there is an abundance of snack foods. Increased weight gain is largely a result not of the amount of calories consumed per meal, but rather of eating more frequently per day.[9]

DIETING DOESN'T WORK

Some weight-loss plans may lead to weight loss in the short term. However, many people don't lose enough weight to be satisfied, and they don't keep it off.

Research shows that the majority of people regain the weight they lose while dieting and that the majority gain back even more weight than they lost. A study found that after two years or more, 83 percent of people gained back more weight than they lost.[10]

One of the main reasons that diets don't work in the long term is because they don't address the root cause of weight gain, which is a disrupted circadian rhythm. Not fixing the root cause of a problem, but simply trying to fix the secondary problems, will solve it only for the short term. Regulating the circadian rhythm through proper timing of exercise, meals, and sleep is the vital and missing piece of information that causes dieters to continually fail in their efforts to maintain their weight loss.

Most weight-loss diets tend to focus more on the calorie content of foods rather than on the nutrient content and satiety level of the food. If food is low in nutritional value and is not satisfying enough, it will leave dieters hungry. The proper foods to eat are those that are nutrient-dense and completely satisfying.

Research shows that dramatically reducing your intake of food increases your risk of binge eating. When you reduce your intake of calories your brain increases its attention to food and develops strong cravings for it. The longer people restrict their food intake, the more they put their attention on food and the more they crave it.[11] This explains why low-calorie diets do not produce lasting weight loss.

Dieting is very stressful. A study found that monitoring calories increase stress levels. Dieting affects psychological well-being and physical health. Therefore, the restriction of calories is ineffective because it increases stress levels and cortisol production—two factors known to cause weight gain.[12] Scientists have known for years that elevated cortisol levels cause weight gain, high blood pressure, and high cholesterol levels, increased risk of heart disease, and increased risk of numerous health problems.

No popular diet plan addresses hidden factors that may hinder or cause unresponsiveness to weight loss. Hidden factors such as hormonal imbalances, blood sugar fluctuations, candida, and psychological issues make it almost impossible to lose weight permanently.

THE CAUSE OF WEIGHT GAIN

All overweight and obese people have a disrupted circadian rhythm, termed *chronodisruption*. Disruption of the circadian rhythm leads to weight gain and a multitude of health problems, such as diabetes and heart disease.

The circadian clock has daily rhythms and coordinates multiple behavioral and physiological processes, including activity, sleep, and eating. All the body's functions are controlled by the circadian rhythm. It is the master clock that manages the other little clocks in the rest of the body. It controls the proper timing of fat burning and fat storing.

All physical functions are synchronized with the rhythmic changes that occur in the natural environment. The health of the body depends largely on how well the circadian clock is working, and how well it's synchronized with the cycles of day and night.

The circadian clock gets disrupted through a high-calorie diet, lack of sleep, excessive light exposure, and improper eating habits (eating late at night, meal timing, meal frequency) which eventually lead to weight gain.[13] [14] [15] Research shows that circadian disruption decreases a person's resting metabolic rate and increases blood sugar levels.[16]

Therefore, to reiterate, the root cause of weight gain and obesity is a disrupted circadian rhythm and it gets disrupted through a variety of improper lifestyle and dietary factors.

RESTRICTIVE DIETS

Diets that work in the short-term damage health in the long term and lead to increased weight gain. For example, the popular high-protein, low-carbohydrate diet increases the production of ketones. A long-term study found that ketogenic diets (high-protein, high-fat, low-carb) lead to changes in beta and alpha cells of the pancreas that regulate the production of insulin and glucagon, which are two hormones responsible for blood sugar regulation. The study found that a ketogenic diet can lead to insulin resistance, fatty liver, a pro-inflammatory state, type 2 diabetes, heart disease, and unhealthy fat regulation, as well as elevated levels of cholesterol, triglycerides, and leptin. Not only that but in the long run the ketogenic diet does not sustain weight loss.[17]

It's common for many people to lose weight, regain weight, and then go on another diet and start the whole process again. The official term for this is *weight cycling*, though it's also known as "yo-yo dieting." Research shows that weight cycling increases the risk of death from all-cause mortality and death from coronary heart disease. Studies find that it's better to maintain a stable weight than to constantly lose weight and gain it back.[18]

One study found that those with weight fluctuations over a period of many years were more likely to die from all-cause mortality than those who were thin and that those who stayed obese lived just as long as those who were thin.[19] Maintaining a stable weight should be the most important priority for those who are unhappy with their weight, but who want to live a long, healthy life.

Constant preoccupation with weight loss and attempts to restrict food intake lead to higher cortisol levels and weight gain. Cortisol, the stress hormone, shortens telomeres, leading to accelerated aging and a lower life expectancy.[20][21]

WHY THE OMAD DIET WORKS

With thousands of fad diets out there, it is becoming increasingly difficult to determine which is effective, which is safe, which is healthy, and which is the most suitable for our individual needs.

The OMAD Diet is effective precisely because it is not another weight-loss program, but rather a scientifically proven weight-management lifestyle plan. Its principles are based on scientific studies that reveal what really works for losing weight and keeping it off. It also provides viable solutions to help those dealing with an extremely difficult or resistant weight-loss problem.

The OMAD Diet seeks to help you address the major cause of weight gain, which is a disrupted circadian rhythm. If you solve the cause of the problem, you will solve the problem permanently.

Recent scientific research shows that restoring the body's circadian rhythm through proper eating habits (meal frequency and timing of meals) and a healthy lifestyle is the key to achieving permanent weight loss as well as dramatically improving health and boosting energy levels.[22 23 24 25]

No matter what you try, if you don't correct a disrupted circadian rhythm, you will not lose weight permanently. Researchers found that those with a disrupted circadian rhythm were unable to lose weight.[26] This explains why some individuals are completely unresponsive to weight-loss programs.

The OMAD Diet provides guidelines that are straightforward and simple, making it easy to follow this lifestyle plan for a lifetime and achieve lasting weight loss.

CHAPTER 1

EATING HABITS

Proper eating habits are the most important factor involved in losing weight permanently. We need to follow the eating habits of our ancestors, the hunter-gatherers, to maintain our health and body weight.

For our ancestors, it was feast or famine. Humans have evolved to endure long periods of time without food. Most cultures around the world eat one, two, or three times per day and do not snack between meals.

People in wealthy, developed countries have access to food whenever they want. This has led people to become "grazers" and to eat whenever they feel like it. Snacking is common and snack foods are readily available.

In recent years, some nutritional experts have recommended grazing or having five or six "mini meals," making people believe that this is a healthy eating habit. However, there are no studies to support this way of eating, and there is actually plenty of evidence against it.

In the short term, eating small, frequent meals every day may help those with hypoglycemia by stabilizing their blood sugar. These people feel good for a while. However, eventually—usually between six and nine months—people notice that they feel hungry all the time. They gain weight and can't seem to lose it.

FREQUENCY OF MEALS

In an effort to combat the obesity epidemic, for many years scientists and medical experts have been trying to find the secret to weight loss. Finally, groundbreaking research has found the answer, and it's so simple that it may easily be overlooked. However, sometimes the simple solutions are the most powerful. Human nature, with its ego, tends to complicate everything, essentially making solutions to problems harder to find. As Albert Einstein said, "Everything should be made as simple as possible, but not simpler."

The secret to losing weight and keeping it off, as well as to improving one's health, is reducing eating frequency.[1] If you get only one thing out of this book, keep this in mind: Eat only once per day and do not have any snacks at all.

Losing weight is as simple as eating only once daily, not consuming any snacks, and skipping dinner (or, if you are hungry, drinking a broth soup for dinner). Once you achieve your weight-loss goal you may decide to have a solid, light dinner eaten two or three hours before bedtime.

In a study comparing two meals per day to six meals per day, researchers found that eating only breakfast and lunch reduced body weight, fasting plasma glucose, C-peptide, and glucagon more than did eating the same amount of food spaced out over six meals. The group eating two meals a day ate their first meal between 6 a.m. and 10 a.m. and the next meal between 12 p.m. and 4 p.m. The group eating six meals per day ate at regular intervals throughout the day. Despite consuming the same number of calories, the group eating only two meals a day lost, on average, three pounds more than the snackers did and about 1.5 inches more from around their waists. The participants eating six meals per day felt less satisfied and hungrier than did those eating only twice per day.[2]

Most cultures around the world eat only two or three meals per day and do not eat snacks. The skinny French and Chinese cultures do not snack at all or do so very rarely.

It is a widespread but scientifically unproven belief that eating small, frequent meals is in some way beneficial. Recent research has found that spreading out food intake into smaller, more frequent meals is associated with weight gain and does not have any beneficial effects on weight or health in the long term.[3][4][5][6] In fact, research shows that eating more than three times a day is a factor that causes weight gain and obesity in the long term.[7]

There is a growing body of scientific evidence to support the health and weight-loss benefits of reduced meal frequency, meal timing, and intermittent fasting. Reduced meal frequency has been shown to suppress the development of various diseases.[8]

The rhythm of eating only once per day around the same time each day teaches the body to experience real hunger followed by fullness and satisfaction. Eating more than three times per day—whether it's a meal, a snack, a sugary drink, alcohol, caffeine, or anything else that raises blood sugar—leads to weight gain.[9][10]

If you are used to eating frequently, slowly work your way down to less frequent eating. For example, start with four meals a day, then work your way down to three, and then two. Finally, if possible, try eating only once per day.

Make the extra effort to sit down, relax, and enjoy each meal. Focus on the food you are eating and on nothing else: no watching television, talking on the phone, standing when you eat, driving, or using a laptop. It may feel strange at first, but you will eat less, digest better, and enjoy your food more.

Once you have reached your ideal weight, you can maintain it effortlessly by eating no more than three times per day and by not snacking.

SUCCESS STORIES

"Until recently, I ate whenever I was hungry and just enough to satisfy my appetite. I guess I was a grazer. I was even making healthy food choices. The problem with my approach is that I was hungry all the time. I would become light-headed and cranky if I didn't get food right away. I've experienced a lot of anxiety around making sure I always had food with me, and I experienced lethargy by the afternoon. After following the advice not to snack at all and to eat only three times per day, my blood sugar and moods have evened out and I've lost weight."

L. Barbeau

"Having tried both ways [eating small but frequent meals and eating less frequently], I've found that eating more meals per day invariably leads to body fat, less of an appetite around meal time, and mood swings. When I eat less often, I lose body fat, and I feel better."

K. Semson

"I am a female trying to lose weight and I also have Polycystic Ovary Syndrome (PCOS), so my hair falls out along with all the other horrid things that come with PCOS. I'm on a super-healthy, low-fat, 1,300-calories-a-day diet. Well, I tried doing six meals a day on a 1,300-calorie diet. I ended up gaining tons of weight and my PCOS symptoms were aggravated. So I know six meals a day is bad!"

Elise K.

"Last year on my doctor's advice I tried six mini meals (200 to 300 calories) every two to three hours. It was hard staying on the schedule. I was constantly focused on eating and food, and never felt satisfied by a real meal. I now eat three regular meals every day. I never starve. This plan helps me be more in tune with my body's hunger signals. Mini meals may work for some, but two to three squares works way better for many. Do what works for you, despite the fads."

Kimber B.

TIMING OF MEALS

Proper meal timing, as well as the amount of calories consumed at each meal, are more important than many people realize. A study found that the best mealtimes are breakfast around 7 a.m., lunch around 12:30 p.m., and a light dinner around 6 p.m. The study also found that breakfast is the most important meal of the day and that skipping breakfast leads to hunger and overindulgence later in the day.[11]

Eating a large, satisfying breakfast every single day has helped dieters reduce their calorie intake throughout the day. Dinner should be the lightest meal of the day and should be eaten at least three hours before bedtime. Dinner must be eaten early, no later than 7 p.m., because people are generally less active in the evening, causing extra calories to turn into fat.

Researchers conducted a 20-week study to examine the effect of meal timing on weight loss. In one group, study participants consumed a breakfast that provided the day's highest amount of calories. In a second group, dinner provided the day's highest amount of calories. Researchers found that having the main meal of the day at breakfast time led to weight loss throughout the 20 weeks and that this effect was independent of total 24-hour calorie intake. A follow-up study done for 12 weeks showed that those who had their main meal and higher calorie intake at breakfast time lost more weight than did those assigned to a higher calorie intake at dinner.[12]

A study found that those who consumed an early lunch (before 3 p.m.) lost 4.85 pounds more than did those who ate lunch later.[13]

Another study found that eating lunch at 4:30 p.m. decreased metabolism and glucose tolerance as compared to a lunch at 1 p.m.[14] Eating an early lunch is the custom in many rural parts of France.

DRINK A SOUP FOR DINNER

Dinner should be the lightest meal of the day. When you are trying to lose weight, skip dinner altogether. If you are really hungry, drink a broth soup or have a liquid meal for dinner. Dinner must be eaten early because people are less active in the evening, and extra calories are more likely to turn into fat.

Most overweight people are unable to estimate proper portion sizes, which results in excessive calorie intake.[15] Therefore, to limit excess food and calorie intake at dinnertime, drink a liquid meal. Studies have found that liquid meals help individuals lose weight.[16][17]

Eating the majority of your calories at breakfast and the least amount of your calories at dinner in liquid form is an effective way to lose weight because fat storage is greatest in the evening.[18]

One of the main reasons the French stay so slim is that they eat very lightly at dinner. The French typically have a very light dinner, with little more than a bowl of soup and a salad. In countries ranking low in rates of obesity, such as Spain and Sweden, residents typically eat their biggest meals at lunchtime. For many Americans, dinner tends to be the biggest and most calorie-dense meal of the day.

Marie Antoinette, the 18th-century French queen (1755-1793) ate cake for breakfast. Butter, milk, and cream were part of her daily diet. However, she stayed slim, with a waist size of 23 inches. She remained slim even after the birth of four children. Her first secret was that she ate only two meals per day. Her second secret was that she ate the majority of her calories during breakfast and lunch, and consumed soup for dinner, a French custom termed "souper."[19]

If eating a big breakfast doesn't suit your lifestyle, you can eat the majority of your calories at lunch. Marie Antoinette indulged her sweet tooth in the mornings, had her main meal consisting of meat or fish and vegetables at lunchtime and then had broth soup for dinner.

Many people wonder why they eat late at night and wake up feeling groggy and run down the next morning. The reason for this is that their circadian rhythms become disrupted when they eat late at night.

In their early development, humans did not have access to food around the clock. They cycled through periods of feast and famine, and modern research shows that this cycling is the way we are meant to eat. By adjusting the timing of when you eat, you can dramatically alter your health and weight.

If you are really hungry, you can consume a high-quality, organic, commercially prepared liquid meal for dinner, or drink a homemade soup made of nothing but vegetables and bone broth (no noodles, rice, or meat). However, you will sleep better and have more energy in the morning if you skip dinner altogether.

The soup that Marie Antoinette drank for dinner is prepared by boiling chicken, turkey, lamb, or beef bones for several hours. The long boiling time releases minerals from the bones. Vegetables such as onion, garlic, celery, kale, chard, and carrots are added, as well as turmeric and herbs, and each bowl contains around 100 calories. The soup can be prepared in advance and frozen in batches that can be quickly reheated when you are tired at the end of a busy day.

HEALTHY EATING HABITS

Properly timing meals and eating less frequently is important for everyone who wants to remain healthy and have energy, not only for people who want to lose weight.

According to the Centers for Disease Control and Prevention (CDC), nearly 90 percent of adults who have prediabetes don't know they have it.

Prediabetes results from eating too frequently and eating high-sugar foods. In 2002, the New York Academy of Sciences published a report stating that all-day grazing can put a person at risk for type 2 diabetes, heart disease, and stroke. The risk increases when insulin spikes after consumption of foods that have high glycemic values. "If you eat only one to two meals a day, your insulin levels have time to even out," says Victor Zammit, head of cell biochemistry at Hannah Research Institute in Ayr, Scotland.

Frequent eating puts pressure on the pancreas, never giving it a rest. When insulin levels are driven again and again many times a day, the pancreas becomes worn out and the cells can become resistant to taking in any more sugar.

The controlled timing of food intake and eating only one meal per day has been found to be the best way to eat if you have diabetes.[20]

In a study by Hanna Fernemark and colleagues comparing a low-fat diet, a low-carbohydrate diet, and a one-meal-per-day Mediterranean diet, it was found that if a person has type 2 diabetes, one massive meal per day is better than several smaller meals. The one-meal-per-day diet included one cup of black coffee for breakfast at 8 a.m. and a large Mediterranean-style lunch at 11:30 a.m. with a glass of wine.[21]

Natural health, Ayurveda, and sports medicine expert Dr. John Douillard states that eating too frequently can result in blood sugar problems, weight gain, and a host of other problems.[22] He explains that when you eat six times a day, you create insulin spikes and, over time, lose the ability to burn fat effectively. This also leads to insulin resistance.

When you eat every two or three hours, your body will burn fuel from those meals or snacks, but it will not burn any of its stored fat for energy. "If you have a healthy snack, like a carrot, in between breakfast and lunch you will burn the carrot but you will not burn any stored fat between those two meals," says Dr. Douillard.

Eating only one to three times per day is essential because, during the five or more hours between meals, the body is forced to burn stored fat.

Whatever you eat turns into blood sugar, so every time you eat, your blood sugar goes up. To keep blood sugar stable, you must eat less frequently.

Insulin is the primary hormone that works to put on fat. By controlling your insulin and keeping it low, you can lose weight. "Eating breakfast, lunch and supper with no snacks in between will provide a natural fast in between meals that will encourage fat metabolism," says Dr. Douillard. After following this eating habit, you will notice "better energy, more stable moods, greater mental clarity, better sleep, fewer cravings and of course, natural and permanent weight management."

For his book *The 3-Season Diet*, Dr. Douillard conducted a study in which he instructed a group to eat three meals a day with no snacks, then measured weight loss and a host of psychological factors. Within two weeks, members of the group experienced better moods, fewer cravings, improved sleep, and less exhaustion after work. They also lost an average of 1.2 pounds per week throughout the two-month study.

INTERMITTENT FASTING

Intermittent fasting has become popular due to the growing research in its favor. Several books have been published on the topic. It typically consists of a very low-calorie allowance on alternate days (ADF) or two days a week (5:2 diet). Normal eating is resumed on non-diet days. It is a simple concept, which makes it easy to follow with no difficult calorie counting every other day. Intermittent fasting works to promote weight loss, but is linked to hunger during the fasting days (very low-calorie days).[23]

Essentially, fasting means eating nothing and drinking only water for a certain period of time. Deliberate fasting is practiced worldwide, mostly for traditional, cultural, or religious reasons. It has been shown that fasting for the biblical period of 40 days and 40 nights is well within the overall physiological capabilities of a healthy adult.[24]

Some believe that intermittent fasting will shift your body into "starvation mode." Starvation mode is a scare tactic that the food and health industry use to keep people fat. However, a study found that there was no change in the metabolic rates of people after 60 consecutive hours of fasting, and even after those 60 hours the reduction of the metabolic rate was only eight percent. Intermittent fasting increases insulin sensitivity. It has been found that intermittent fasting is more effective for weight loss than is traditional calorie restriction.[25]

Fasting is a powerful detoxification method, proven to remove toxins from the body.[26] The scientific term for detoxification is autophagy. Autophagy means that your body flushes out everything it doesn't need. This happens at the cellular level. Cells consume their defective parts. Autophagy is essential for detoxifying cells and guaranteeing their proper function. If we eat all the time, our cells never get a chance to detoxify and rebuild themselves. Cells cannot break down defective parts and absorb materials to build new cell parts at the same time, so fasting for certain periods is essential to encourage the process. Research reveals that when animals and people are allowed to eat as they please, very little autophagy occurs. Even a tiny snack is enough to stop this process of cellular repair.[27 28 29 30] In the absence of this important repair mechanism, defects in the cell can accumulate, causing disease and accelerated aging.

There is a large body of research to support the numerous health benefits of fasting.[31 32 33 34] Fasting reduces the risk of type 2 diabetes, cardiovascular disease, cancer, and neurodegenerative disorders.[35 36 37 38 39 40 41 42 43 44] Fasting has also been proven to delay aging and increase lifespan. Many people carry out fasting in conjunction with intestinal cleansing through enemas or colonics to increase the healing effect that fasting provides.[45 46]

There is significant empirical and observation-based evidence that medically supervised fasting spanning periods of 7 to 21 days is effective in the treatment of chronic diseases such as rheumatic diseases, chronic pain syndromes, hypertension, and metabolic syndrome.[47]

Fasting also improves thinking ability, depression, insomnia, and anxiety. Gabriel Cousins, MD states, "I often observe in the fasting participants that by four days of [full-day] fasting, concentration seems to improve, creative thinking expands, depression lifts, insomnia stops, anxieties fade, the mind becomes more tranquil and a natural joy begins to appear. It is my hypothesis that when the physical toxins are cleared from the brain cells, mind-brain function automatically and significantly improves and spiritual capacities expand."

Abstaining from food for even one full day (24 hours) is difficult for some people and not suitable for everyone. There are different types of fasts and different ways to abstain from food for a period of time. You can improve your health and lose weight without taking on full-day fasts. Fasting overnight might have similar benefits to full-day fasts.[48]

By eating only once per day and eating as much as you want at that time, you can take part in fasting without going hungry. For example, by eating breakfast at 7 a.m. or eating lunch at 1 p.m. and by not eating dinner (except for a broth soup if you feel hungry), you are fasting from 1 p.m. until 7 a.m. the next day, which is 16 hours of fasting. If you don't eat for 12 to 16 hours, your body will go to its fat stores for energy. You will then break the fast with "break-fast."

CONTROL INSULIN TO BURN FAT

The cells of the body need sugar for energy. However, sugar cannot get into most cells directly. After a meal, a rise in blood sugar levels signals cells in the pancreas, called beta cells, to secrete insulin, which pours into the bloodstream.

Insulin signals cells to absorb sugar from the bloodstream. Within 20 minutes after a meal, insulin rises to its peak level. If there is more sugar in the body than it needs, insulin helps store the sugar in your liver.

In healthy people, two to three hours after a meal, insulin levels return to a baseline and the pancreas makes a different hormone called glucagon. This hormone tells your liver to release the sugar it has stored to sustain your blood sugar levels. Just as insulin signals the fed state, glucagon signals the starved state. It serves to mobilize glycogen stores from the liver when there is no food intake.

Gluconeogenesis typically begins four to six hours after the last meal and becomes fully active as stores of the liver's glycogen are depleted. It's during gluconeogenesis that your body will burn your stored fat for fuel.[49]

If you eat a snack or another meal within six hours of eating, insulin rises again, which inhibits fat burning. You are supposed to get a snack between meals, but it should come from your fat stores, not from the consumption of food. Eating a large dinner or eating after dinner makes matters even worse because sleep is a prime opportunity to burn fat.

When the body is fed every two to three hours, it uses fuel from those meals instead of burning its fat stores. The body adapts to being fed constantly without needing to dig into its fat stores. However, when you eat one or two meals a day and don't snack in between, the body is forced to burn its fat. "If you snack just as your insulin blood level is decreasing, it will promptly rise, even if you have a good snack such as fruit and nuts," says Eduardo Castro, MD, a specialist in fat-loss resistance syndrome. Eating frequently keeps insulin levels elevated constantly, which makes your body continually store fat.

High insulin levels inhibit the body's fat burning ability. You must keep insulin secretion low. Low levels of insulin allow your body to produce large amounts of lipase, the hormone responsible for releasing fat into your bloodstream to be used as fuel.[50]

You want to finish eating each meal within an hour or less and not eat your next meal until six or seven hours have passed. This means not eating or drinking anything that will prompt insulin release until your next meal. Caffeine, tea, a sugary drink, or a small snack will prompt insulin release.

If you drink coffee, tea, freshly squeezed fruit juice, or any beverage besides water, consume them during meals, not in between meals. Commercially prepared fruit juices such as apple juice or orange juice are the worst, as they are very high in sugar and quickly raise blood sugar levels.

If you have problems with digestion (gas, bloating, burping, low energy after eating), drink bone broth or lacto-fermented beverages with your meals. They assist in the digestion and assimilation of nutrients.

EAT LESS OFTEN

Eating only once per day and consuming absolutely no snacks will not only help you lose weight permanently, it will dramatically improve your health.

A groundbreaking study compared the weight and health effects of two groups of people eating the same high-calorie diet. One group ate only three times per day, while the second group ate more frequently and consumed snacks. The group that ate frequently accumulated belly fat and developed nonalcoholic fatty liver disease, while those eating only three times per day did not. The study suggests that snacking contributes to weight gain and nonalcoholic fatty liver disease. This study surprisingly reveals that those eating a high-calorie diet in only three meals do not experience the negative effects on their health or weight that people eating more frequently do.[51]

Another study found that eating during specific times (time-restricted feeding) decreases body weight, lowers concentrations of triglycerides, glucose, and low-density lipoprotein (LDL) cholesterol, and increases concentrations of high-density lipoprotein cholesterol.[52]

Scientists have discovered that reduced meal frequency can prevent the development of diseases and increase the lifespan of laboratory animals.[53 54]

If you are unable to eat less frequently because of gnawing hunger and cravings for food, there are hidden health factors that you need to address (see Chapter 5).

A HIGH-FAT DIET

The U.S. Department of Agriculture (USDA) noted in 2013 that fat consumption has declined in the United States in the last few decades, but rates of obesity have not gone down.

Surprisingly, recent research has found that it's not so much what you eat, but when you eat it. Disruption of circadian rhythms by eating ad libitum (eating at any time of the day) is the problem that leads to obesity and metabolic disorders. The circadian clock regulates the expression and activity of certain metabolic enzymes, hormones, and transport systems.

Time-restricted feeding limits the time and duration of food availability (meal frequency). A study found that mice confined to specific time-restricted periods of eating a high-fat diet became leaner and healthier than mice that ate the same diet but ate whenever they wanted. The mice on the time-restricted feeding schedule consumed an equivalent amount of calories from a high-fat diet as did those with unlimited access, yet were protected against obesity, hyperinsulinemia, fatty liver, and inflammation.[55]

Mice fed a time-restricted, high-fat diet had much better satiation, 18 percent lower body weight, 30 percent decreased cholesterol levels, 10 percent reduced TNF-levels (tumor necrosis factor involved in systemic inflammation), and improved insulin sensitivity as compared to the group of mice fed a low-fat diet, ad libitum. This is very interesting because the amount of calories per gram of food was higher in the high-fat diet. The time-restricted, high-fat diet group had no caloric restrictions, yet lost more weight than did the mice fed a low-fat diet, ad libitum.[56]

In another study of a structure similar to that of the previously mentioned study, time-restricted feeding caused less weight gain than did all-hour food access for mice eating a high-fat, high-sugar diet over 12 to 26 weeks. Interestingly, time-restricted feeding of a high-fat diet actually led to weight loss of up to 12 percent when applied to mice that were already obese.[57]

This recent groundbreaking research can help us understand why the French eat rich, fatty foods like bread, butter, dessert, and pâté, but stay thin—they don't snack between meals. The French adhere to specific mealtimes and don't typically eat between mealtimes. They consider snacking between meals to be overindulgent and unnecessary for adults.

PREVENTING TYPE 2 DIABETES

Type 2 diabetes is a metabolic disorder characterized by the inability of pancreatic beta cells to secrete enough insulin to maintain normal blood sugar levels.

You can conduct two tests to analyze your risk for type 2 diabetes and to check for prediabetes. Without intervention, prediabetes is likely to become type 2 diabetes in 10 years or less. You want to regularly check your fasting glucose with a blood sugar monitoring device called a Fasting Glucose Test. This is a blood sugar sample taken when you first wake up in the morning. The result is a great screening number because blood sugar tends to be higher in the morning, and this is one of the first indicators of rising blood sugar. To stay out of the danger zone in terms of diabetes risks and associated degenerative health concerns, keep in mind that the safe range for blood sugar is between 70 and 85 mg/dL (milligrams per deciliter). You can also check your blood sugar two hours after a meal. Healthy blood sugar two hours after a meal should be lower than 125mg/dL.

Hemoglobin A1c measures the percentage of glycated hemoglobin in one's blood. Hemoglobin A1c levels should be below 5.6 percent.

Eating too frequently puts a strain on the pancreas. When the pancreatic beta cells are working nonstop, there is a risk of type 2 diabetes. Loss of first phase insulin secretion is an independent predictor of type2 diabetes.[58]

Irregular eating patterns appear to produce a degree of insulin resistance.[59] It is beneficial to stay consistent with the timing of meals every day.[60]

If you are overweight and have type 2 diabetes, reduce your eating frequency to lose weight and increase insulin sensitivity. Space your meals five, six, or even seven hours apart, and eat each meal around the same time every day. A study found that eating only breakfast and lunch helps lower BMI in people with type 2 diabetes. After 12 weeks, researchers found that those who ate breakfast and lunch and no dinner lost an average of 1.23 points off their BMIs. The study concluded that, for people with type 2 diabetes, eating fewer, larger meals may be more beneficial than eating more frequent meals.[61]

Do not consume snacks, alcohol, or coffee between meals. Caffeine raises insulin levels and impairs glucose metabolism in those with type 2 diabetes. It's best to limit your caffeine intake if you have diabetes.[62 63 64] If you want to enjoy a cup or two of coffee, consume it during meals.

If you experience hunger before your next meal, you will need to improve your diet and eat low glycemic index (GI) meals that do not elevate insulin levels rapidly. Rapid elevation of insulin levels produces feelings of increased hunger and the desire for more food.[65]

When you don't eat between meals, the pancreas has time to recharge and prepare for efficient insulin release for the next meal. The liver has time to generate energy and deplete its stores of glycogen.

MAKE IT WORK

If you are used to eating frequently and snacking, it is suggested that you gradually improve your eating habits. Start by eating only four meals a day, four hours apart, and work your way down to three meals. Eventually, work your way down to only one solid meal a day and if you are really hungry only drink a bone broth soup for dinner.

Children, teenagers, young adults, bodybuilders, and athletes, or those with an exceptionally fast metabolism, are able to eat more frequently without gaining weight. However, with age, their eating habits will likely catch up to them, and they can develop health issues related to bad eating habits such as snacking and eating frequently.

The following testimonial comes from the book, *Secrets from the Eating Lab*, and attests to eating only two meals per day. When he was younger, a man had raised a pig for the state fair. He fed his pig only twice per day, allowing the pig to eat as much as it wanted during its two meals. His friends fed their pigs the traditional way, letting the pigs have access to food all day long and allowing them to eat whenever they wanted. When it came time for judging, the man's pig had grown to be very lean, strong, and healthy, while his friends' pigs had grown fat.

Pigs are not known for their lean figures; therefore, the man who had raised the lean pig, who himself was overweight, was convinced that he had found the secret to losing weight and keeping it off. He decided to eat only twice per day. He ate as much as he wanted and ate whatever he wanted, but he ate only twice per day. He lost 42 pounds in two years and has kept it off for seven years and counting.

As easy as the eating less frequently sounds, each individual is unique and will have to find a way to make this strategy work for his or her situation and lifestyle. Time, work schedule, willpower, and other factors need to be considered. For some, it's very difficult to eat only once per day, and they need two or three meals. However, three meals should be the maximum amount of meals allowed.

If you have issues with willpower, cravings, late-night eating, or emotional eating, it is important to get rid of any quick cooking devices, such as a microwave, in your kitchen and to keep absolutely no food in the kitchen. Simply prepare meals ahead of time and keep them in your freezer to be heated up in the oven. If you can afford it, eat out at restaurants offering healthy food and leave your fridge and freezer empty.

Human nature always looks for the easy way. By creating barriers that demand a substantial amount of time and effort, you can reduce the motivation to eat frequently. Do not keep food on hand that you can eat right away. If food is not there or is hard to access, you are less likely to eat it.[66]

Preparing meals ahead of time on weekends and freezing them also works for people who have a limited amount of time during the week. If you can afford it, you can save plenty of time by having organic, healthy, freshly prepared meals delivered to your door every week and you can keep them in the freezer to be eaten only once per day.

LOSE WEIGHT FAST

To lose a significant amount of weight (up to one pound per day) in a fairly short amount of time (one to six months), eat only once per day and consume only low glycemic index (GI) and low glycemic load (GL) foods.

Eating one low GI meal per day is the most effective method of losing weight fast. When you eat, your pancreas releases insulin, but between meals, your pancreas releases glucagon. Insulin promotes the storing of calories, while glucagon promotes the release of stored calories.

High GI foods promote weight gain. If you eat a meal that contains mostly high glycemic foods (sugar, white rice, white bread), your blood sugar level will skyrocket. Your body won't be able to break it down fast enough and therefore will store it as fat. Low glycemic foods promote satiety, minimize insulin secretion, and lead to weight loss.[67]

Eating only once per day is a form of intermittent fasting, as you are skipping two meals and consuming only one large meal. If energy (in the form of recently consumed food) isn't available, the body will be encouraged to draw from its fat reserves.

Although some may worry about the body entering starvation mode, contrary to popular belief, intermittent fasting involving 16- to 24-hour periods of no food consumption has been shown to actually increase the body's metabolic rate, leading to a greater rate of fat loss.[68] Resting energy expenditure increases in early starvation.[69] Resting energy expenditure is the number of calories you burn if you rest all day.

A study found that despite consumption of the same number of calories, participants lost weight when eating only one meal per day as compared to three meals per day. Fat mass was significantly reduced and lean body mass tended to be greater after eight weeks of one meal per day.[70]

Throughout history, people would (and many cultures still do) eat only one or two meals per day. The Romans ate only one meal per day in the middle of the day. "The Romans believed it was healthier to eat only one meal a day. They were obsessed with digestion and eating more than one meal was considered a form of gluttony," explains food historian Caroline Yeldham.

The best time to eat your one meal is at lunch like the Romans did. You can also try making breakfast or dinner the time when you eat your only meal. Experiment with different times when you eat your one meal to see what works for you. Everyone is different, but the principle is the same: eat only once per day.

When eating your one meal, eat as much as you feel like, until you're completely satisfied. You can do a full-course meal consisting of a soup, entrée, main course, and dessert.

The pages of this book could be filled with testimonials about the power of eating less frequently to lose weight, but since you need to try it for yourself before you believe it, here are some testimonials with the most impressive results.

Des O'Connor, an English comedian, broadcaster, and singer, was asked how he stayed slim, vibrant-looking, and virile at age 70. He explained that he eats only one meal per day, and, in fact, eats as much as he wants during that one meal. He swears by this eating habit and has followed it for over 40 years. He is a strong believer in the fact that using excess energy for digestion (eating all the time) only depletes the energy that the body requires for healing.

Adam Minsky, a young man weighing 230 pounds, reported that he lost 51 pounds in four months by eating only once per day. He's tried various diet plans, such as Atkins,

South Beach, Weight Watchers, Jenny Craig, and many others, but found that eating only once per day works like nothing he's tried before. In one week he lost six pounds and in the first month, he lost 15 pounds. In four months, he lost 51 pounds. One year later, he had maintained his weight loss.

Herschel Walker, a former professional football player, eats only one meal per day at dinner and started when he was 18 years old. He does not eat breakfast or lunch. He drinks only water during the day. He is in phenomenal shape and looks much younger than he is.

SUCCESS STORIES

"I went from 363 pounds to 197 pounds. I had only one meal per day and no snacks or anything with calories. I ate whatever I wanted. You'll find that you crave healthier foods as time passes and your stomach shrinks. Don't worry about that now. Just no junk food. Eat one average-sized plate completely filled up. It regulates blood-sugar levels and metabolism. This is why this plan works when others do not. There is a reason why every culture the world over has historically had fasting as an integral part of their regimens. It helps the mind and body."

Samson

"I have lost 18 pounds in four weeks simply by eating one meal per day. I am proof that it works! I eat my big meal at lunch and even being a diabetic I can pretty much eat whatever I want, except processed sugars. I do only 30 minutes of elliptical about three days a week."

K. Schmorr

"People who eat one meal a day do it for its many health benefits and to stay in the fat burning zone, increase good cholesterol, balance blood sugar and, most importantly, promote longevity. It is best to eat a balanced amount of protein, healthy fats, and carbs from vegetables. Avoid eating three to four hours before going to sleep. This diet is not for children and teenagers who are still developing, but it is for adults who are overweight, and those looking to stay fit and healthy and to live longer."

S. Sehjal

"The only way I've ever successfully lost weight is by eating one meal per day. When I tried eating three to six small meals, I was hungry all the time, didn't sleep well, and gained weight. When I eat one big meal per day, I have more energy, don't feel hungry, and sleep well. The first time I ate one meal per day, I lost 15 pounds, losing one pound per week. Now I have to do this about once or twice per year, for five to seven weeks, to maintain my weight."

G. Becker

"This has been the most successful diet I've ever tried. I have lost 41 pounds eating only one meal a day. I used to eat six small meals a day, go to the gym, and exercise every day. Nothing worked better for me than eating only one meal a day."

D. Fowler

"I've lost 10 pounds in 17 days. It really hasn't been that hard to eat only one meal a day. I don't deprive myself. I eat anything I want; I simply eat it only once per day. I'm less hungry during the day than I was when I ate all day long. To prevent myself from getting hungry during the day, I stay busy, drink lots of water, and don't nibble. I have found that the more I eat, the more I want to eat. My energy level is good even though I don't eat during the day. If I need energy, I drink a 5-Hour Energy drink."

Tony G.

"The great thing about eating only once a day is that I can eat whatever the family eats. Nothing fancy, nothing out of the ordinary, just regular food. Nothing is off limits. I think the obvious key to this diet is that you can eat whatever you want once a day to the point of being pretty full; as long as you don't seriously overdo it and gorge yourself during your one meal, you will lose weight. I found it way too hard to eat rabbit food multiple times a day with only one or two cheat meals on the weekend. This is truly the best way: Eat what you want only once a day and still lose weight. Simple, and much easier than 'mainstream' diets. I think one of the best things about this diet is that you can adapt it to suit your lifestyle. Here is how I do it: I'm eating my meal in a very short window of 30 minutes, I eat enough to feel full, I finish with something sweet, like a piece of chocolate, and I eat anything and everything I want. There are certain things I avoid, like sodas."

Dave M.

"I have been eating one meal a day for four months and I have lost 45 pounds. I have been on every single diet out there and this is the only one that's worked for me. I can't stick to any diet longer than a week, but by eating one meal a day, I get to eat my favorite foods. Since losing 45 pounds I have noticed a dramatic difference in my health."

Anna

"I lost 20 kilograms in four months. This worked so well because I promised myself I could have three courses every day if I wanted: soup, a main course, and dessert. I think this is an ideal diet for me, as there is only one rule: Eat whatever you want just once a day."

Amy S.

"I have realized that the only way the one-meal-a-day diet works for me is to fast until mealtime. I can't take anything in the day, not even coffee or tea, because I drink my coffee with sugar and tea with honey, and I think this spikes my blood sugar and I want to eat. So I fast until my main meal and I drink only water during the day."

Calypso

"I have been having one meal per day and I've lost 85 pounds in six months without starving myself and I have been eating a delicious, fulfilling meal every day. I'm motivated because I can still enjoy a meal I truly enjoy every single day. I'm losing weight by eating whatever I want!"

Jose

"Eating one meal a day is the only thing that has ever worked to help me lose weight. In only a few months, I have lost 25 pounds. I intend on eating only one meal a day for the rest of my life because I have the body I want without obsessing over calories."

Elle D.

"I have tried everything. For years I have struggled with dieting. I couldn't deal with the restriction and felt like I would be fat forever. I started eating one meal a day for three months and I have effortlessly dropped 33 pounds. I have never been successful with losing weight, never been able to lose more than a few pounds. What amazes me is that once I got used to the diet, I never felt hungry. The best thing is the freedom I feel. No calorie counting, no packing snacks to work, and no planning out what I need to eat every day."

Cindy

"For one year, I ate only one meal a day. This is the only method of dieting that I can follow for the long term. It's really not much of a diet, but a lifestyle. I have lost over 70 pounds in a year."

Mary F.

"It is important for our metabolism to have extended periods of not eating or eating very little. We are not designed to have constantly elevated levels of glucose

in the blood, nor are we designed to have the repeated spikes in insulin which are created by frequent eating, especially eating high glycemic index foods. I lost 42 pounds by eating only one meal a day. I drew myself back from the early stages of insulin resistance and have never felt better."

A. MacDowell

"I started eating one meal, once a day, four months ago. At the beginning, I didn't think this diet would work for me, but it does. It takes some willpower at first, but after the second week, you get used to it. I have lost 46 pounds in four months and I will continue eating once a day until I'm at my ideal weight. I was very overweight and I can honestly say this diet has saved my life."

S. Farrell

SKIP DINNER

The old adage by nutritionist Adelle Davis—"Eat breakfast like a king, lunch like a prince, and dinner like a pauper"— stands up to the test of research. Eating an indulgent, high-protein breakfast increases satiety, metabolism, and energy levels.

Skipping breakfast or eating late at night causes weight gain and leads to higher fasting insulin, total cholesterol, and LDL cholesterol.[71][72][73][74][75][76] You are better able to metabolize food during the day when you are awake and active. Food eaten right before bedtime or during the night will likely be converted into fat.

The circadian clock plays an essential role in regulating body weight because it has a strong influence on metabolism and how the body handles fat and sugar.[77][78][79] When a person's circadian clock is thrown off by eating at the wrong time, it can, over time, contribute to weight gain.

Dr. Fred W. Turek has demonstrated that mice with a mutation in the brain's suprachiasmatic nuclei responsible for synchronizing circadian rhythm had a disrupted feeding pattern. The mice ate more at all hours of the day. The mice were obese and had a number of metabolic problems, including high cholesterol and high blood sugar.[80]

Numerous scientists have found that it is important to properly time caloric distribution across the day to maintain weight loss. People with a high caloric intake during breakfast with plenty of protein lose more weight and keep it off than do those with a high caloric intake during dinner.[81] Eating breakfast regularly is so significant that it has been shown to protect against weight gain, despite a person's daily calorie intake.[82]

A big, nourishing breakfast rich in protein also has many health benefits. It reduces the risk of type 2 diabetes and cardiovascular disease.[83][84] It has been shown to enhance cognitive performance.[85] It improves glycemic control in those with type 2 diabetes.[86] A study demonstrated that lower levels of GL and higher portions of protein intake at breakfast were associated with higher levels of energy.[87]

EAT THE RIGHT BREAKFAST FOODS

Milk is promoted as a healthy beverage. Pasteurized cow's milk and products made with cow's milk are commonly consumed during breakfast. However, research shows that pasteurized cow's milk is a very unhealthy choice, associated with obesity, atherosclerosis, diabetes, cancer, and neurodegenerative diseases.[88]

The processed, factory-farm-produced milk we drink today is not like the raw, organic milk our ancestors drank. Growth hormones and estrone found in factory-farm cow's milk promotes weight gain. Growth hormones and estrone are also found in protein powder containing whey protein.[89]

If you want to lose weight and improve your health, you must eat the right foods for breakfast. A healthy breakfast consists of eggs, legumes, nuts, seeds, fish, and poultry. If you include dairy in your breakfast, consume only raw, grass-fed, organic milk from cows, goats, or sheep. If you drink a protein shake, consume only non-dairy protein powder, such as pea and hemp protein.

EAT DESSERT AT BREAKFAST

Extremely high-calorie intake will always play a role in obesity, and there is no way to avoid this fact. However, to achieve permanent weight loss, it's important not to restrict yourself. Restrictive diets that ban desserts or delicious treats are likely to fail because at some point you will give in to your cravings.

If you feel like eating cake or other sweet desserts, the best time to indulge is at breakfast. The body's metabolism is most active in the morning and you have the rest of the day to burn off the calories.

In a study of clinically obese adults led by Daniela Jakubowicz, MD, two groups of study participants ate the same number of calories per day. The only difference was the number of calories consumed at breakfast.

Group one ate 1,085 calories a day. Their smallest meal was breakfast, consisting of 290 calories. Group two ate 1,240 calories a day. They ate breakfast as well as a dessert, consisting of 610 calories. Lunch was 395 calories and dinner was 235 calories. After 16 weeks, both groups lost approximately the same amount of weight. After completing the diet, study participants were told to continue the diet, but were allowed to eat more if they were hungry.

The first four months of the eight-month study focused on weight loss, while the last four months focused on weight maintenance. In the first four months, the small-breakfast eaters lost an average of 28 pounds, while the big-breakfast eaters lost an average of 23 pounds. After eight months the small-breakfast eaters regained 18 pounds while the big-breakfast eaters lost an additional 16.5 pounds.

Jakubowicz explains that having an indulgent breakfast including dessert helps reduce cravings and hunger during the day. The group that had a smaller calorie breakfast reported higher hunger cravings throughout the day, leading to overeating and weight regain. The group that consumed a big breakfast and dessert experienced few if any cravings during the day.[90]

Attempting to avoid sweets entirely can create a psychological addiction to these foods in the long term, explains Jakubowicz. Having dessert during breakfast can control cravings for the rest of the day.

There are two pointers to keep in mind when having dessert for breakfast. The dessert should be sweetened with stevia, lo han guo, erythritol, or xylitol rather than with white sugar. It's also important to eat a high-protein breakfast.[91] As long as you follow these two pointers you will lose weight by eating dessert during breakfast, as it will likely cause you to eat less during the day.

If you want to enjoy a cup of coffee with your cake or dessert during breakfast, drink your coffee black. The bitter taste of coffee beans complements the sweetness of cake or other desserts very well. Try to get used to drinking your coffee black, with nothing added to it.

If you must sweeten your coffee, use stevia, lo han guo, erythritol, xylitol, or raw Manuka honey. If you want to add milk or cream to your coffee, use organic, raw, grass-fed milk or cream from goats or sheep instead of pasteurized cow's milk.

Having dessert and drinking coffee are simple pleasures that many people enjoy. As long as you understand the importance of meal timing, you can enjoy coffee, dessert, and high-fat foods just like the French do.

PORTION VS. CALORIE DENSITY

Contrary to standard advice to eat smaller portions, it's better to eat low-calorie-density foods. Research shows that people eat a fairly consistent amount of food on a day-to-day basis.[92] [93] We all have to eat a certain amount of food to feel comfortably full every day—usually between two and three pounds a day.[94] This finding holds true whether the amount of food contains many calories or only a few calories.

If we eat less than the amount we're used to eating every day, we tend to feel hungry and deprived. Therefore, cutting back on the amount of food you eat per day is an approach that won't work in the long run. If you feel hungry and deprived all the time, eventually your willpower will crumble.

A much better approach is to eat the same amount of food you're used to but to eat foods high in nutrients and low in calorie density. That way you can eat satisfying portions of food and feel full while reducing calorie intake.

Research found that eating satisfying portions of low-calorie-density foods is a more successful strategy for weight loss than is portion control.[95][96]

Calorie density is the amount of energy or calories in a particular weight of food. Generally, it is the number of calories in a gram. Foods with a lower calorie density provide fewer calories per gram than do foods with a higher calorie density. The lower the calorie density of the food, the more you can eat of it. For example, two ounces of chocolate contains 240 calories. To eat the same amount of calories in lettuce, you would have to eat 3.2 pounds of lettuce.

Diets consisting of foods low in energy density were shown to result in weight loss.[97][98][99]

You don't want to make calorie counting a religion, but try to keep within your calorie requirement range by eating mainly foods that are very low in calories per gram. You can easily look up your daily calorie intake requirements online by searching for "Estimated Energy Requirement," or use the Harris Benedict formula to estimate your daily caloric needs with respect to your average activity level.

Most overweight people have a sedentary lifestyle that includes only light physical activity associated with typical day-to-day living. The more active you are, the more calorie-dense foods you can consume.

Sedentary women between the ages of 19 and 30 need no more than 2,000 calories per day. Sedentary women between the ages of 31 and 50 need no more than 1,800 calories per day. Sedentary women older than 51 need no more than 1,600 calories per day.

Sedentary men between the ages of 19 and 30 need no more than 2,400 calories per day. Sedentary men between the ages of 31 and 50 need no more than 2,200 calories per day. Sedentary men older than 51 need no more than 2,000 calories per day.

Calorie density is measured by the gram, so a food's calorie density tells you how many calories are in one gram of that food. To calculate calorie density from food labels (calories per gram):

1. Get the calorie count.
2. Get the weight of the serving in grams.
3. Divide the calorie count by the weight.

The emphasis should be on the types of food that can be eaten in satisfying portions instead of on reducing the portion sizes. If you select foods that are low in energy density, you will be able to eat your usual amount of food. This will help eliminate the sense of deprivation that can accompany calorie restriction.

Foods Low in Calorie Density

Long-grain brown rice

Wild rice

Red snapper

Yogurt

Whole wheat pasta

Turkey breast

Boiled sweet potato

Cod fish

Cottage cheese

Shrimp

Light tuna

Whole milk

Soba buckwheat noodles

Foods High in Calorie Density

Chocolate

Bacon

Potato chips

Peanut butter

Doughnuts

Cheesecake

Swiss cheese

Whole wheat crackers

Cheddar cheese

Popcorn

Mayonnaise

Vegetable oil

You don't need to eliminate high-calorie-dense foods completely from your diet, but simply eat smaller portions when you do eat them. The key to long-term weight loss is not restricting any food or drink unless absolutely essential (e.g., because of allergies or food sensitivities).

Whether eating at a restaurant or at home, pause in the middle of your meal and sip on a cup of coffee or tea for about 10 to 15 minutes. After taking a break from eating, see if you are feeling hungry. You may find that you are full after the first half of your meal and that you don't feel the need to eat the rest of it.

Start all your meals (breakfast and lunch) with a soup. In Japan, miso soup is served with every meal. Studies show that consuming a low-energy-dense soup before eating leads a person to eat less of his or her main meal.[100] [101] Those who had soup before their meals ate 20 percent less. This reduction in food intake did not lead to increased hunger or decreased fullness at the end of the meal.[102]

You can also eat fruit or low-energy-dense salad before—rather than during or after—your main meal. Research has found that consuming fruit or salad before a meal can enhance satiety and reduce the amount of food a person eats during his or her main meal.[103] [104]

Many people digest fruit better on an empty stomach, and nutrition experts and holistic doctors recommend eating fruit on an empty stomach rather than after meals. This is because fruit digests so quickly (typically within 30 minutes of eating) and when eaten on a full stomach could cause fermentation, gas, and bloating.

FOOD ADDICTION AND CRAVINGS

What stops people from eating healthier and lower in calorie density is their addiction to certain foods and their desire for flavor and good taste. However, the biggest misconception about losing weight and eating healthier is that you have to eat only fruits, vegetables, low-fat, low-carb, and low-sugar.

A healthy, balanced diet means eating whole foods rich in nutrients. You can eat grass-fed meat, wild-caught fish, free-range eggs, grass-fed dairy, low GI sweetened desserts, and a huge range of low-GI whole grains made into fresh bread, muffins, cookies, pancakes, cakes, chips, pizza, and other delicious baked goods. You just need to know where to purchase high-quality foods and ingredients and how to make them into delicious meals, desserts, and baked goods.

If you are highly addicted to certain unhealthy junk foods, start eating better gradually. Over time, as you get healthier, you will crave healthier foods.

Start by making subtle changes that your taste buds will not notice. If you are addicted to sugar and desserts, replace white sugar with raw honey, stevia, lo han guo, erythritol, or xylitol. If you are addicted to salt and salty snacks, replace table salt with Celtic and Himalayan sea salt.

Thanks to numerous healthy substitutes (see Appendix A) available from health food stores, you can replace every single unhealthy food with a healthy alternative.

EAT DESSERT AND LOSE WEIGHT

If you love to eat sweets and cake, then natural sweeteners like raw honey, coconut palm sugar, stevia, lo han guo, erythritol, and xylitol are your best friend.

Using natural sweeteners instead of sugar to sweeten all desserts is such a simple way to reduce weight gain caused by the excessive consumption of sweets. If every bakery, cake maker, chocolate maker, and candy manufacturer used stevia instead of sugar, then obesity would not be such a crushing problem. Dieting or dietary restrictions would not be necessary, and you could eat dessert at each meal if you really had a desire for it.

Lo han guo is an exotic fruit extract that has zero calories and zero glycemic impact, making it safe for diabetics and hypoglycemics to use.[105] Lo han guo can be used in your baking as a sugar substitute.

Xylitol is just as sweet as table sugar (sucrose) but has about 40 percent fewer calories and 75 percent fewer carbohydrates. Xylitol also won't raise your blood sugar like regular sugar does, as the body does not require insulin to metabolize xylitol.[106]

Raw honey is a good sugar substitute, has a low glycemic response, and is suitable for those with diabetes.[107] Raw, unprocessed honey has antioxidants, minerals, vitamins, amino acids, enzymes, and phytonutrients. It is considered a superfood. It is good for sweetening tea, coffee, or drinks. Pasteurized honey has a higher GI, so always use raw, unheated honey.

Blackstrap molasses contains a variety of nutrients, such as manganese, copper, iron, calcium, potassium, magnesium, vitamin B6, and selenium. Refined white sugar and corn syrup are stripped of virtually all nutrients except simple carbohydrates. Blackstrap molasses has a GI of 55.

Coconut palm sugar has a lower GI (35) than does white sugar. It is rich in magnesium, potassium, zinc, and B vitamins. In terms of taste, out of all the natural sweeteners, it comes closest to white sugar. It's good for baking and sweetening coffee, tea, or smoothies.

Raw sugarcane juice has a low GI. It has no simple sugars and doesn't cause blood sugar to soar like white sugar does. It contains calcium, magnesium, potassium, iron, and manganese.

Lucuma powder is made from whole Peruvian lucuma fruit. It is rich in minerals such as iron, zinc, potassium, calcium, magnesium, vitamin B3, and beta carotene. Lucuma has a low GI and GL.

Stevia comes in powdered or liquid form. It's a good substitute for white sugar when baking. Stevia is sweeter than sugar, so you need less of it. It has no effect on blood sugar levels. It has a GI of zero, and it has zero calories.

Pure, organic maple syrup is an excellent source of manganese and antioxidants. It also contains riboflavin, zinc, magnesium, calcium, and potassium. Pure maple syrup has a GI of 55.

CHAPTER SUMMARY

- Eat once per day, with no snacks, caffeine, or drinks between meals except for water and unsweetened, caffeine-free drinks that will not affect blood sugar. If you can't eat only once per day, eat a maximum of two or three times per day.

- Eat your one meal a day at the same time every day. Space your meals five to six hours apart if you eat two or three times per day. For example, have breakfast at 7 a.m., lunch at 12:30 p.m., and dinner at 7 p.m.

- Ideally, eat your one meal a day at breakfast time. If this doesn't suit your lifestyle, eat your one meal a day at lunch, ideally before 3 p.m.; the earlier, the better.

- If you are hungry, drink a liquid meal or have only broth soup for dinner; better yet, skip dinner completely.

- Utilize intermittent fasting by fasting overnight. By eating only once per day and eating as much as you want during that one time, you can fast without going hungry.

CHAPTER 2

DIET

The foundation of a healthy diet is consuming low GI and low-GL foods. Studies show that low GI and low GL diets promote weight loss.[1] Although low-carbohydrate, high-protein diets have become popular means of losing weight, there is a large body of evidence that indicates low GI diets are the best way to lose weight and prevent diseases such as diabetes and cardiovascular disease.[2]

A HEALTHY DIET

Most weight-loss diets are unbalanced and unhealthy, eliminating certain foods or food groups (carbs, protein, fats) that are essential to long-term good health. The only foods a person should eliminate from his or her diet are those they can't tolerate (e.g., cow's milk because of allergic reactions, or gluten because of celiac disease).

Carbohydrates, fats, and protein are all important components of a balanced, healthy diet. A good rule of thumb is to divide your plate in the following way at each meal: one-half vegetables, one-quarter protein, and one-quarter whole grains or starches. In other words, 50 percent veggies, 25 percent protein, and 25 percent whole grain or another healthy starch.

According to extensive research into the healthiest cultures, the ideal diet consists of mainly organic produce, whole grains, pulses, seeds, nuts, fish, meat, and dairy. It also entails the avoidance of foods detrimental to one's health, including sugar, white flour, and foods not suitable for a person due to allergies or other individual factors.

It is important to consume a variety of whole foods and not eat the same foods day after day. It is important to vary your diet to make sure you are covering all your nutritional bases. It may be possible for some people to develop intolerances to foods eaten too often. For example, some people have developed food sensitivities to their favorite foods because they ate them on a daily basis for long periods of time.

Most studies show that reducing healthy fats is harmful. Some people think that they are doing their health good by replacing butter with margarine and by eliminating eggs and red meat from their diets. However, Dr. Weston Price found that the world's healthiest cultures ate protein in the form of organ meats and dairy products and considered animal fats absolutely essential to good health.[3] Their diets consisted of healthy fats, meats, fruits, vegetables, legumes, nuts, seeds, lacto-fermented foods, bone broth, and whole grains in their whole, unrefined state, as well as some raw foods of both animal and vegetable origin.[4] This is what a healthy, balanced diet should be composed of. Dr. Price found that people eating this diet were free of disease, dental decay, and mental illness. When they started to consume an unhealthy, typical Western diet, their health rapidly deteriorated. He found that consumption of refined grains, canned foods, hydrogenated fats, refined oil, sugar, and pasteurized milk spoils our God-given inheritance of physical perfection and vibrant health.

HUNGRY FOR CHANGE

Everyone who wants to lose weight, feel better, have more energy, and get healthier should watch the documentary *Hungry for Change* (2012). The documentary discusses the real cause of weight gain and why diets don't work. It exposes shocking secrets the diet, weight loss, and food industries don't want you to know. Some of the key points are:

- Diets do not work. Ninety to ninety-five percent of people who go on a diet will not only regain their weight but gain back even more.

- Foods in modern societies are high in calories and low in nutrients. On the other hand, in healthier traditional cultures, whole foods are high in nutrients and generally low in calories.

- Many people in America are chronically overfed but undernourished. Being chronically starved of nutrients causes a person to constantly eat in an effort to fulfill their body's requirements for nutrients.

- People in modern societies are not eating real, whole foods, but rather food-like products such as boxed, packaged, canned foods, weight loss drinks, and food bars.

- Many packaged foods are now touted as having zero calories, no fat, and no sugar. However, this is simply a marketing ploy. For example, foods marketed as low-fat can contain plenty of sugar, and sugar converts easily into fat. Foods marketed as having zero calories and no sugar typically have many toxic artificial sweeteners that cause weight gain in the long run.

- Food companies are similar to tobacco companies. They know that if they addict a customer, they have that customer for life. Consequently, they use various chemicals that are known to cause addiction: monosodium glutamate (MSG), processed sugar, and artificial sweeteners. They put chemicals in their food so that people keep buying it.

- Artificial sweeteners such as aspartame are very toxic and contribute to weight gain in the long run.

- Diet soda has zero calories, but because it contains artificial sweeteners, studies have shown that within a few years, you will be fatter than when you first started drinking diet soda.

- Don't get products labeled "low fat." It's not fat that makes you fat, but rather sugar that makes you fat. Sugar gets converted straight to body fat. The body needs healthy sources of fat to stay healthy. If you're on a low-fat diet, you'll constantly be hungry because you need the correct amount of fat to feel satiated. You need healthy fat from avocados, organic extra virgin coconut oil, ghee, and nuts.

- Insulin is the fat-producing hormone. Insulin takes the excess sugar you ingest and puts it into your muscles. As soon as the muscles' energy stores are full, the excess sugars are converted into fat. Avoid foods that quickly convert to sugar in your body such as white bread, white flour pasta, white potatoes, muffins, waffles, pancakes, cereal, and white rice.

- Sugar is a drug as addictive as cocaine. White sugar should be illegal. Processed foods, especially sugar, kill more people than all drugs combined.

- White flour, white sugar, and high fructose corn syrup are all like cocaine—whitened, extracted, refined products taken from a natural product and made into an addictive product. Sugar and high fructose corn syrup can be found in everything. They are in pasta sauces, juice, cereal, salad dressing, and nearly every boxed, packaged food.

- MSG is one of the worst ingredients found in many packaged, boxed foods, as well as in restaurant food. It's found in about 80 percent of modern food products. MSG is almost impossible to avoid. When scientists want to make a mouse fat, they give it MSG. MSG has many names; many even sound natural, and that's why sometimes it's hard to spot when you look at food labels. It can be called glutamic acid, yeast extract, hydrolyzed protein, bouillon, broth stock, malt extract, gelatin, soy protein, whey protein, and natural flavors. MSG is very dangerous because it excites the brain, causing a chemical reaction that results in addiction.

- It can be hard to get enough vegetables in your diet. Vegetables are the most hated food group and yet are the most important. Although vegetables are best consumed in their whole forms, the easiest way to get your full required serving of vegetables is to juice them along with some sweet fruits to make the juice palatable. Most people are overfed and undernourished; by juicing vegetables with fruits, they get a highly concentrated source of nutrients that are easy to digest and taste good.

- Many of the food labels in grocery stores are deceptive; that's why you want to buy and eat whole foods, not processed, packaged, boxed foods.

- If you're upset, don't eat. That's because you're not fully aware of what you're putting in your body. People overeat when they are stressed, upset, angry, and frustrated.

THE WESTON PRICE DIET

Dr. Weston Price and his wife traveled around the world in search of the secret to health. He investigated some of the most remote areas of the planet. He observed excellent health in many native cultures who ate specific foods. He found that their health rapidly declined once they began consuming unhealthy foods such as sugar, alcohol, processed grains, pasteurized dairy, and packaged foods. Incomplete development of the face and body, crooked teeth, and disease became common.

The comprehensive research of Price as documented in his masterpiece book, *Nutrition and Physical Degeneration*, is unfortunately largely ignored in a country where saturated fat and cholesterol from animal sources are condemned. Through his extensive research, Dr. Price discovered that non-industrialized people do not gain weight on their traditional diets.

All traditional cultures consume some sort of animal protein and fat from fish and other seafood; water and land fowl; land animals; eggs; milk and milk products; reptiles; and insects. Primitive and traditional diets have a high food-enzyme content from raw foods such as raw dairy products; raw meat and fish; raw honey; fruits; and naturally preserved, lacto-fermented foods.

Total fat content of traditional diets varies from 30 percent to 80 percent. Traditional diets contain nearly equal amounts of omega-6 and omega-3 essential fatty acids.

The diets of healthy primitive and non-industrialized peoples contain no refined or denatured foods such as refined sugar or corn syrup; white flour; canned foods; pasteurized, homogenized, skim, or low-fat milk; breakfast cereal; packaged foods; commercially prepared fruit juice; soft drinks; soy milk; tofu; refined or hydrogenated vegetable oils; protein powders; artificial vitamins; or toxic additives and colorings.

Dr. Price does not recommend low-fat diets, diets that restrict fat, vegetarian diets, or vegan diets. Dr. Price makes the following dietary guidelines on his website (http://www.westonaprice.org):

- Do not practice veganism; animal products provide vital nutrients not found in plant foods.

- Eat only organic meat and eggs. Avoid factory-farmed meats and eggs.

- Avoid highly processed luncheon meats and sausages containing MSG and other additives.

- Avoid rancid and improperly prepared seeds, nuts, and grains found in granolas, quick-rise bread, and extruded breakfast cereals, as they block mineral absorption and cause intestinal distress.

- Avoid canned, sprayed, waxed, bioengineered, or irradiated fruits and vegetables.

- Avoid artificial food additives, especially MSG, hydrolyzed vegetable protein, and aspartame, which are neurotoxins. Most soups, sauce mixes, and commercial condiments contain MSG, even if they're not labeled as such.

- Seeds, grains, and nuts should be soaked, sprouted, fermented or naturally leavened to neutralize naturally occurring antinutrients, such as phytic acid, enzyme inhibitors, and tannins.

- Eat organic poultry, beef, lamb, game, organ meats, and eggs as well as wild-caught fish and seafood.

- Eat whole, organic milk products from pasture-fed animals, preferably raw and/or fermented, such as whole yogurt, cultured butter, whole cheeses, and fresh and sour cream.

- Use only healthy fats and oils, including butter and other animal fats, and organic extra virgin coconut oil.

- Eat fresh fruits and vegetables, preferably organic, in salads and soups, or lightly steamed.

- Prepare homemade meat stocks from the bones of chicken, beef, lamb, or fish and use liberally in soups and sauces.

- Use unrefined Celtic sea salt and a variety of herbs and spices for food interest and appetite stimulation.

- Make your own salad dressing using raw apple cider vinegar and expeller-expressed flax oil.

- Use natural sweeteners such as raw honey, maple syrup, and stevia powder.

- Consume only unpasteurized wine or beer in strict moderation with meals.

- Cook only in stainless steel, cast iron, glass, or good-quality enamel.

The body needs a rich supply of the fat-soluble vitamins and fat-soluble activators found in animal fats. Many of the vitamins and minerals found in vegetables cannot be absorbed without fat, and protein cannot be assimilated without fat. The body will rob its own stores of fat-soluble vitamins to digest protein if a sufficient amount of fat is not consumed with it, leading to nutritional deficiency.

Dr. Price recommends a diet consisting mainly of freshly ground, soaked, and fermented whole grains; grass-fed bone marrow; rare-cooked, organic, grass-fed meat; organic, grass-fed organ meats; raw eggs; wild, uncooked fish; fish eggs; seafood; nuts; seaweed; grass-fed yellow butter; grass-fed cream; tomatoes; raw/unpasteurized organic milk from grass-fed cows; and green vegetable juices made from such veggies as parsley, cilantro, zucchini, and cucumber.

To provide the body with fat-soluble vitamins he suggests making a daily smoothie with two raw eggs, one cup raw milk or kefir with two to four ounces raw cream along with some stevia for sweetness. In addition, half a teaspoon of fermented cod liver oil is taken with a quarter teaspoon "high-vitamin butter oil" two to three times daily with meals.

THE MEDITERRANEAN DIET

The Mediterranean diet is one of the best ways of eating for maintaining a healthy weight and preventing disease.[5] It has been shown to prevent age-related weight gain.[6][7]

A study found that the Mediterranean diet was much more effective in weight reduction than a low-fat diet. Weight reduction among participants after two years was six to nine pounds for the low-fat group and nine to thirteen pounds for the Mediterranean-diet group.[8]

Healthy fats, which are staples of the Mediterranean diet, keep you feeling fuller longer than do diets that restrict or forbid fat altogether. Monounsaturated fats are found in nuts and avocados. Polyunsaturated omega-3 fatty acids are found in fatty fish (salmon, mackerel, and halibut).

According to Dr. Demosthenes Panagiotakos and Christina-Maria Kastorini, MSc, PhD, the Mediterranean diet is not only the best way to eat to lose weight, but also the best way to prevent disease. The diet is associated with lower risk for cardiovascular disease, type 2 diabetes, obesity, and some types of cancer. A 10-year study found that following a Mediterranean diet was associated with a decrease in early death rates by over 50 percent.[9]

Many people want to lower their cholesterol with diet alone. The Mediterranean diet has been shown to be a very effective method of lowering cholesterol levels and reducing heart disease risk. It's also a good alternative to drug therapy.

In combination with the Mediterranean diet, fish oil, and soluble fibers—such as psyllium, oat bran, guar gum, and pectin—have been shown to reduce cholesterol levels in multiple studies.

The lipid-lowering benefits of fish have been well known since epidemiologists noticed that the Greenland Inuit have a low coronary mortality. They eat a high-fat, high cholesterol diet, but one rich in fish, especially those containing the omega-3 fatty acids EPA and docosahexaenoic acid (DHA). It is suggested that eating two or three fish per week will prevent coronary disease. Herring, mackerel, sardines, salmon, and anchovies are especially rich in omega-3 fatty acids.[10]

An even larger reduction in heart disease death was found among people who took fish oil capsules (900 mg omega-3 per day) instead of eating fish. Fish oil is especially effective at lowering elevated very low-density lipoprotein (VLDL) and chylomicron levels. Fish oil has antithrombotic, anti-arrhythmic, and anti-inflammatory properties in addition to lipid-lowering effects.[11]

THE GLYCEMIC INDEX

The GI was developed by Dr. David J. Jenkins at the University of Toronto during research to discover which foods were best for people with diabetes.

The GI is a numerical system of measuring how rapidly a particular food turns into sugar and how much of a rise in circulating blood sugar it triggers. With foods numbered from 1 to 100, the closer a number is to 100, the higher the GI and the more it affects blood sugar levels. The lower the GI number, the less the food affects blood sugar levels.

Foods with a GI of 55 or less are considered low, while values of 56 to 69 are medium. Those 70 or higher are high GI values. Pure glucose serves as a reference point and is given a GI of 100. High-glycemic foods are between 70 and 100 on the index and include white bread or bagels; white sugar; russet potatoes; melons; pineapple; corn and rice pasta; macaroni and cheese; corn flakes; instant oatmeal; whole wheat bread; bran flakes; puffed rice; pretzels; rice cakes; popcorn; and soda crackers.

Foods with a high GI make a person's blood sugar levels rise rapidly, which can increase the person's chance of getting diabetes. They also make managing type 2 diabetes a challenge. Foods with a low GI release glucose more slowly and steadily into the bloodstream and therefore have the lowest insulin response.

If blood sugar rises too quickly, the pancreas secretes a greater amount of insulin. Insulin helps bring sugar out of the bloodstream, primarily by converting the excess sugar to stored fat. High blood sugar leads to greater insulin release and more storage of fat. It is important to eat low GI foods to prevent weight gain and type 2 diabetes.

Research provides compelling evidence that high GI foods increase the risk of obesity. In one study, rats were split into high- and low-GI groups over 18 weeks. Rats fed the high-GI diet were 71 percent fatter and had eight percent less lean body mass than did the low GI group.[12]

Overweight or obese people consuming low GI and low GL foods lost weight and had decreases in body mass, total fat mass, BMI, total cholesterol, and LDL cholesterol as compared to those consuming a low-calorie, low-fat diet. Study participants lost more weight even though they could eat as much as they desired. Researchers concluded that lowering the GL of the diet appears to be an effective method of promoting weight loss and improving lipid profiles.[13] Minimizing the consumption of high GI foods is truly one of the easiest ways to reduce your weight.

Scientific evidence has shown that individuals who followed a low-GI diet over many years had a lower risk of developing type 2 diabetes, coronary heart disease, and age-related macular degeneration.[14]

Try to avoid foods high on the GI. If your favorite food has a high GI, combine it with a low GI food to reduce the GL of the meal. Fat, protein or fiber tend to lower the GI value of the food, as they all slow the entry of sugar from a particular food into the bloodstream.

The complete list of the GIs and GLs for more than 1,000 foods can be found in the article "International tables of GI and glycemic load values" in the Diabetes Care Journal.

The GL takes into account not only how quickly a certain food is converted into sugar in the body, but also how much sugar a particular food contains. The GL multiplies the GI of a certain food by the carbohydrate content of the actual serving. A GL of 20 or more is high, a GL of 11 to 19 is medium, and a GL of 10 or less is low.

It is best to know the GI and the GL of a particular food to decide if you want to eat it. For example, the sugar in carrots and watermelon is readily absorbed into the bloodstream; therefore, they are both ranked high on the GI. People might decide to avoid carrots and watermelons because they assume that because they are high on the GI they will cause weight gain. However, although the sugar in carrots and watermelons is absorbed into the bloodstream quickly, they don't have much sugar, so they have a low GL. This explains why even though they are high on the GI, you will not gain weight eating small portions of them.

THE SATIETY INDEX

Researchers from the University of Sydney performed an interesting study in which they compared the satiating effects of various foods. The results of the study clearly indicated that certain foods are much better than others for satisfying hunger. The researchers concluded that the satiety index is useful for the treatment and prevention of overweight and obesity.[15]

The satiety index measures different foods' ability to satisfy hunger. The most satisfying foods they tested were plain boiled potatoes, brown pasta, oatmeal, fish, and meat. People who consumed these foods were less likely to feel hungry immediately afterward. Foods that did the worst job of satisfying hunger were croissants, donuts, candy, and peanuts.

The satiety index is a valuable tool for those wanting to lose weight. "A diet which simply recommends cereal for breakfast overlooks the fact that muesli is only half as satisfying as porridge [oatmeal]," says Susanna Holt, PhD. "Many health-conscious dieters will eat a meal based on several pieces of fruit and some rice cakes and then wonder why they feel ravenous a few hours later. These kinds of extremely low-fat, high-carb meals do not keep hunger at bay because they are not based on slowly digested carbs and probably don't contain enough protein. A dieter would be better off eating a wholesome salad sandwich on wholegrain bread with some lean protein like tuna or beef and an apple. This kind of meal can keep hunger at bay for a very long time."

You can find the satiety index in the article "A satiety index of common foods" in the September 1995 European Journal of Clinical Nutrition or online in PDF format.

YOU ARE WHAT YOU EAT

The common saying, "you are what you eat" is evident among all those with a "good diet" and a "bad diet." Nutrition researchers and health experts have consistently shown the dramatic difference a good diet has on a person's physical appearance, energy levels, health, and weight.

Physician and nutritionist Robert McCarrison discovered that ancient Indian races such as the Sikhs and certain Himalayan tribes had good physical development, health, hardiness, and endurance thanks to their good diet. Their diet consisted of coarsely ground whole wheat, unpasteurized milk, unpasteurized milk products, tubers, roots, green leafy vegetables, fruit, and, occasionally, meat.

McCarrison conducted an experiment on rats entitled "A Good Diet and a Bad One: An Experimental Contrast." This study reveals the health effects of the typical American diet (white bread, margarine, sugar, food preservatives).[16]

Some rats were fed a "good diet" designed to resemble that eaten by the Sikhs and consisting of whole wheat flour, uncooked vegetables, fresh fruit, sprouted legumes, butter, fresh whole milk, and, occasionally, fresh meat. Other rats were fed a "bad diet" designed to resemble that eaten by many Western people and consisting of white bread made from American white flour; vegetables cooked in water to which pinches of sodium bicarbonate and common salt were added; a butter substitute; processed, tinned meat; packaged jam; sugar; and common food preservatives. McCarrison showed that the rats fed a "good" diet for six months were physically efficient, healthy, strong, and active, while the rats fed the "bad" diet for six months were physically inefficient, weak, low in energy, and sick.

In his book, *Nutrition and Physical Degeneration*, Dr. Price documents his travels to various isolated parts of the earth where the inhabitants had no contact with civilization. While there, he studied their health and physical development. In every isolated region he visited, Price found tribes in which or villages where virtually every individual displayed physical perfection and an almost complete absence of disease—even those living in physical environments that were extremely harsh. He presented photographs in his book of primitive tribes who had a high degree of physical perfection, as well as beautiful, straight, white teeth with no decay (as compared to the teeth of "civilized" people whose diets of sugar, refined grains, canned foods, pasteurized milk and devitalized fats and oils caused facial deformities, tooth decay, and disease). The diets of the healthy "primitives" Price studied consisted of unpasteurized milk, butter, cream, cheese, dense rye bread, bone broth soups, seafood, fish, oats, fish liver, fish roe, seal oil and blubber, wild game meat, organ meat, glands, marrow, whole grains, tubers, vegetables, and fruits.

HEALTHY SUBSTITUTES

You can easily sabotage your weight loss efforts if you frequently binge on extremely high-calorie foods and high-calorie-dense foods (four to nine calories per gram), including baked and regular potato chips, croissants, cookies, French fries, pretzels, cake, and many other high-sugar foods.

If you have intense and frequent cravings that you can't control, you need to address hidden factors (see Chapter 5). Chromium deficiency is common in North America and may cause intense cravings for sugar. Candida overgrowth and parasitic infection can also cause intense hunger and constant cravings for certain foods; they are hidden factors in weight gain and an inability to lose weight no matter what you do. About 3.5 billion people suffer from parasite infections of one type or another.

If you get cravings for certain high-calorie-dense junk or snack foods, replace them with healthier substitutes that are similar in taste and texture and lower in calorie density.

Carob is a good replacement for chocolate. It has a similar texture and flavor but, unlike chocolate, is lower in calories, higher in calcium, and higher in fiber, and has no dairy, caffeine, or theobromine. Carob is naturally sweet-tasting, so many carob bar brands do not add sugar. Carob is also a great substitute for chocolate if you have allergies or sensitivities to chocolate. You can find carob bars at health food stores or online.

For cookies, cupcakes, donuts, muffins, pancakes, waffles, brownies, cakes, pies, and all other desserts and baked goods, you can substitute a few ingredients to make these desserts healthier and lower in calorie density. The two main ingredients to eliminate are white flour and white sugar, as both have high glycemic values, causing blood sugar control problems and weight gain.

Replace wheat flour with coconut flour, quinoa flour, oat flour, spelt flour, kamut flour, rye flour, barley flour, or buckwheat flour. Coconut flour is a popular choice. It is high in fiber, low on the GI, and gluten-free. Oat flour is another popular choice. It tastes a lot like white flour but is much healthier. It's lower on the GI and is a rich source of soluble fiber.

Replace white sugar with low GI, natural sweeteners such as pure stevia, coconut palm sugar, sugarcane juice, maple syrup, Manuka honey, and blackstrap molasses. Not everyone reacts to these sugars the same way, even if they are low in the GI, so it's best to buy a glucose meter and test your blood sugar before and after eating one of these sweeteners to see which works best for you.

Agave syrup has become popular in recent years, but it's not a good choice. The Glycemic Research Institute announced that it has stopped all future clinical trials of agave as a result of the latest clinical trials, in which diabetic subjects experienced severe and dangerous side effects related to the consumption of agave. The institute also legally de-listed and placed a ban on agave for use in foods, beverages, chocolate, and other products. Manufacturers that produce and use agave in products are warned that they can be held legally liable for negative health incidents related to ingestion of agave.

Homemade vegetable chips are good substitutes for potato chips when you are craving something crispy and salty. You can make oven-baked chips out of kale, sweet potatoes, butternut squash, beets, eggplant chips, spinach, Brussels sprouts, radishes, and zucchini. The most popular are oven-baked kale chips.

When you're craving French fries and a burger you can replace white potatoes with sweet potatoes and a regular burger with a healthier version.

French fries made from white potatoes do not offer many nutrients. They are high in starch and calories. On the other hand, sweet potato fries are packed with calcium, potassium, and vitamins A and C, and are high in fiber. They are also comparably low in calories. Homemade, oven-baked, sweet potato fries have a taste and texture that's similar to regular potato fries. Sweet potatoes are loaded with beta-carotene, which is what gives them their bright orange color. Frying is the worst way to cook sweet potato fries because it adds unnecessary calories and depletes nutrients, so make sure to oven bake them.

For a healthier and lower calorie version of regular burgers, use spelt or kamut hamburger buns, organic grass-fed goat cheese, and organic 100-percent grass-fed beef patties or free-range turkey patties. If you can't locate grass-fed meat patties in your area, buy them online and have them delivered to your door. There are numerous organic farms that accept orders online or by phone.

CARBOHYDRATES

Carbohydrates have gotten a very bad rep in recent years. However, the main problem is not carbohydrates in themselves, but the type of carbohydrates consumed. High-glycemic carbohydrates produce weight gain. Low-glycemic carbohydrates do not produce weight gain and are essential to good health. China and Japan have very low obesity rates. These populations eat large amounts of low-glycemic carbohydrates (up to 78 percent of their calories) and citizens remain slim throughout their lives.

Carbohydrates are part of a balanced, healthy diet. Low-glycemic carbohydrates are an important source of essential nutrients such as thiamin, riboflavin, niacin, and folate, as well as iron, magnesium, and selenium. Low-glycemic carbohydrates are also rich in dietary fiber. Dietary fiber lowers the risk of coronary heart disease, stroke, hypertension, diabetes, obesity, and certain gastrointestinal diseases.[17]

The best times to consume larger amounts of carbohydrates are when you first wake up and before and after workouts, as you can be sure that you will put them to use and burn them off, not store them as fat.

PROTEINS

Meat and dairy are important sources of protein and nutrients. The only protein sources that should be avoided are processed meat products, as well as deep-fried and smoked meats.[18 19 20]

People subsisting mostly or entirely on vegetables and fruits have teeth containing caries, bone problems, and tuberculosis.[21] In a survey of 1,040 dentists and their wives, those who had the fewest health problems and the fewest diseases had the most protein in their diets.[22]

Studies of the Soviet Georgian people show that those who consumed the most meat and fat in their diets lived the longest.[23] Masai and kindred African tribes' diets consist mainly of milk, blood, and beef. Their members are free of heart disease and have low cholesterol levels.[24 25]

The indigenous Okinawa islanders have one of the longest life expectancies on the planet. A typical Okinawan lives for about 110 years of a healthy, productive life. The most important factor influencing their longevity is the food they eat. They eat generous amounts of pork and seafood and do all their cooking in lard.[26]

The Japanese, who have one of the longest life spans of any nation, eat moderate amounts of eggs, pork, chicken, beef, seafood, organ meats, and fish broths.

The people of southern Indian who are vegetarian have one of the shortest life spans in the world.[27] Animals considered strictly vegetarian consume insects that adhere to the plants they eat.

Animal protein is the best source of protein and fat-soluble vitamins. Isolated protein powder or vegetable protein is inferior in quality. Protein powder made from soy, whey, casein, or eggs are made by a high-temperature process that denatures the protein, causing it to have nitrates and other carcinogens. Soy protein is high in phytates that block mineral absorption, phytoestrogens that depress the thyroid, and enzyme inhibitors that cause cancer.[28]

The amount of protein needed by each person varies. Some people require a lot of protein, while others do not produce enough hydrochloric acid in their stomachs to handle meat intake very well.

FATS

Healthy fat is essential, helping to absorb calcium as well as vitamins A, D, E, and K. Saturated fats are claimed to be the main causes of heart disease, but studies have shown that trans fats (vegetable oils, margarine, processed foods) are the main culprits. Trans fats cause diabetes, cancer, and cardiovascular diseases.[29]

Heating unsaturated fats cause them to become toxic and harmful. All hydrogenated and partially hydrogenated oils have been overheated. To prevent disease, avoid all margarine, shortening, foods containing partially hydrogenated vegetable oil, pastries, and fried and deep-fried foods.[30]

Vegetable oils (canola oil, soybean oil, sunflower oil, corn oil, safflower oil, sesame oil, sunflower oil, palm oil), when heated, are detrimental to one's health and raise the risk of cardiovascular disease.[31]

Vegetable oil and foods that contain partially hydrogenated oils can't be extracted simply by pressing or separating naturally. They must be chemically removed, deodorized, and altered. They become toxic because they are chemically altered, yet they get promoted as healthy.

Butter, lard, and animal fats are highly stable and do not form dangerous free radicals when heated. Extra virgin coconut oil and ghee (clarified butter) are also stable when heated.

High-quality seed oils such as flaxseed, hempseed, and sesame seed oil should be cold-pressed and organic, and can be used as ingredients in homemade salad dressings or added when cooked foods have cooled. They should never be heated, as they form dangerous free radicals when heated.

Diets of healthy, native peoples around the world are rich in saturated fats; these people don't have heart disease and cancer. Modern day researchers fail to take into account other dietary factors of people who have heart disease and cancer. Some researchers claim a link between consumption of meat/saturated fat and heart disease and cancer, but fail to take into account other dietary factors, such as trans fats, white flour, and sugar consumption.

Protein and fat occur together, and this is the way they should be eaten. Protein cannot be properly utilized without fat. A high-protein, low-fat diet may be touted as effective for weight loss, but in the long run, it causes health problems and nutritional deficiencies.

Eating a diet too low in fat can interfere with the absorption of fat-soluble vitamins A, D, E, and K. The body needs fat to utilize these vitamins. Consuming low-fat milk, egg whites, and lean meats can lead to nutritional deficiencies.

Saturated fats such as coconut oil, ghee, and butter are acceptable for use in cooking at higher temperatures. Monounsaturated fats such as olive oil are best used in salads and not heated. Polyunsaturated fats such as vegetable, seed, and nut oils should not be heated or used in cooking.

There is little evidence to support the claim that a diet low in cholesterol and saturated fat reduces deaths from heart disease. Interestingly, research found that people who ate the most cholesterol, the most saturated fat, and the most calories weighed the least and had lower serum cholesterol.[32]

Coronary heart disease is rare among Polynesians who eat a high-saturated-fat diet. In Britain, a Medical Research Council survey also showed that men who ate butter ran half the risk of developing coronary heart disease as compared to those who ate margarine. Eggs have a very high cholesterol content. Most doctors still tell patients to eat no more than about three eggs per week. Dr. Uffe Ravnskov conducted his own test of this theory by eating a total of 59 eggs over nine days. His cholesterol fell by more than 11 percent, from 7.23 mmol/L (millimoles per liter) to 6.39 mmol/L. Careful analysis of the available research, including randomized trials, indicates that, contrary to widespread opinion, lowering cholesterol levels does not appear to be an effective way of reducing cardiac death.[33]

Processed foods, sugar, and white flour are the problem, not fats and proteins in their natural, raw, organic states. "The introduction of food processing with the Industrial Revolution in the 19th century and the use of chemical additives and other processes in the 20th century is the only satisfactory explanation for the dramatic changes in incidence of vascular disease in the 20th century," explains Kilmer McCully, MD.

In a 10-year study of fat and numbers of heart events, researchers found that only polyunsaturated fats significantly increased heart disease.[34] Vegetable fat consumption is linked to high rates of cancer, but animal fat is not.[35]

Margarine is marketed as "heart healthy" but is actually harmful and should be completely avoided. In one study, researchers found that diets containing fats solely of animal origin coincided with little heart disease or diabetes, but diets that contained margarine and vegetable oils coincided with high levels of heart disease and diabetes.[36] Research has concluded that oxidized plant sterols found in margarine may be a contributor to heart disease.[37] Instead of margarine, use yellow, organic, grass-fed butter and ghee, and pure, unrefined, organic extra virgin coconut oil.

TOXIC FOOD AND BEVERAGE

Seneca, a Roman philosopher, said, "Men do not die, they kill themselves." This is true today, as many people consume foods that are detrimental to their health. Even some natural foods are best avoided due to their naturally high toxin content.

Canned, boxed, and frozen foods have no enzymes. Even raw foods may be enzyme deficient if they are picked before they are ripe. Enzymes develop only when a plant ripens in the soil. Irradiating food or treating it with preservatives can also destroy enzymes. Food lacking enzymes are not digested properly and putrefy in the colon.

Packaged meals contain MSG. MSG in the body has been linked to strokes, nervous system infections, and a large number of diseases, such as lupus, cancer, chronic hepatitis, and neurodegenerative diseases.[38]

All processed foods contain low amounts of potassium and high amounts of sodium. Max Gerson, MD, a German physician who cured cancer and other diseases nutritionally, believed that excess sodium is a major cause of cancer. He believed that the entrance of sodium and the loss of potassium in cells initiates disease. To prevent cancer, Gerson recommends keeping potassium levels high and sodium levels low in the body.

Aflatoxins are toxic metabolites produced by certain fungi on foods. Research has shown that aflatoxins can cause liver cancer.[39 40]

Peanuts contain the fungus Aspergillus flavus and its mycotoxin, aflatoxin. Corn and edible mushrooms also have high levels of poisonous and carcinogenic fungi.[41] Research has found that corn consumption is associated with death from cancer of the esophagus and gastric cancer.[42 43] Studies show that mushroom consumption can induce cancer.[44]

Commercially stored grains also develop mycotoxins. Researchers found an association between esophageal cancer and patients who consumed stored grains.[45]

Brewer's yeast has been shown to cause breast cancer. Products containing brewer's yeast include bread, muffins, cakes, pies, pastries, and cookies. It is best to avoid all commercially prepared baked goods.[46]

Puffed wheat, puffed oats, and puffed rice found in products such as rice cakes, corn flakes, and some boxed cereals are toxic. The pressure of the puffing process produces chemical changes, turning a nutritious grain into a poisonous substance that has caused rapid death in animals. A laboratory study showed that rats that were given puffed wheat died within two weeks. Autopsies revealed that the rats had dysfunction of the pancreas, liver, and kidneys and degeneration of the nerves of the spine, all signs of insulin shock.[47]

Boxed cereals that have extruded grains at high temperatures and pressures to make flakes and shapes should be avoided. Extruded whole grains have even more adverse effects on blood sugar than do sugar and white flour.[48]

Soy has been found to interfere with the functioning of the thyroid gland, cause thyroid problems, and interfere with the utilization of iodine. Excessive soy intake has been reported to be responsible for the development of goiters.[49]

Soybeans contain anti-nutrients (lectins, saponins, oxalates, enzyme inhibitors, phytates). Phytic acid reduces the bioavailability of vitamins A, B12, D, and E and the minerals calcium, zinc, magnesium, and iron, creating the potential for nutritional deficiencies in people who consume a lot of soy foods. Traditional preparation techniques (soaking, fermenting, and heating) reduce the anti-nutrients contained in soy.

Moderate amounts of traditionally prepared and minimally processed soy foods may offer some health benefits.[50] [51] However, there are health risks associated with the consumption of non-fermented soy, highly processed soy, and soy protein isolate found in certain protein powders.[52]

If you choose to consume soy, make sure to consume only properly prepared soy that has been soaked, fermented, and heated.

White vinegar contains acetic acid, which causes anemia and cirrhosis. These vinegars are found in pickled foods. On the other hand, apple cider vinegar contains malic acid, which has beneficial effects on health.[53]

Alcohol consumption is linked to many illnesses.[54] Research has found that alcohol consumption increases the risk of certain cancers.[55] A study of more than one million middle-aged British women concluded that for every additional drink regularly consumed per day, the incidence of breast cancer increased by 11 per 1,000.[56] Binge drinking of four to five drinks increased the risk of breast cancer by up to 55 percent.[57]

Everyone should remove soft drinks and diet sodas (marketed as low-calorie, zero-calorie, and sugar-free) from their diets. Plenty of research clearly shows that regular soda consumption leads to weight gain, nutritional deficiencies, type 2 diabetes, hypocalcemia, cavities, high blood pressure, and other health problems.[58]

A study found that sugar-sweetened beverages and artificially sweetened beverages were both linked to an increased risk of type 2 diabetes.[59] Another study found that those who consumed sugar-free, zero-calorie diet soda containing artificial sweeteners were more likely to gain weight in the long term than were those who consumed naturally sweetened soda.[60]

The San Antonio Heart Study examined 3,682 adults to study the effects of long-term consumption of artificially sweetened drinks. The study participants were followed for seven to eight years and their weights were monitored. After adjusting for common factors that contribute to weight gain such as dieting, exercise, or diabetes status, the study showed that those who drank artificially sweetened drinks had a 47-percent higher increase in BMI than those who did not.[61]

The American Cancer Society conducted a study of 78,694 people who were the same in regard to age, ethnicity, socioeconomic status, and health. At a one-year follow-up, 2.7 percent to 7.1 percent of those who were more regular users of artificial sweeteners had gained weight as compared to those who didn't use artificial sweeteners and who were matched by initial weight.[62]

The Nurses' Health Study found that eight-year weight gain in 31,940 women was linked to the use of artificial sweeteners.[63] The National Heart, Lung, and Blood Institute Growth and Health Study followed 2,371 girls for 10 years. Both diet and regular soda drinking was associated with increased BMI.[64]

SUGAR IS POISON

High sugar intake increases advanced glycation end products (AGEs), which are sugar molecules that attach to and damage proteins in the body. AGEs speed up the aging of cells, which may contribute to a variety of chronic and fatal diseases.[65]

Sugar produces a rise in triglycerides, a leading cause of heart disease.[66] Sugar feeds cancer cells and has been connected to the development of cancer of the breast, ovaries, prostate, rectum, pancreas, biliary tract, lung, gallbladder, and stomach.[67 68 69 70 71 72] Sugar can also cause arthritis, multiple sclerosis,[73 74] diabetes,[75 76] osteoporosis,[77] Alzheimer's disease,[78] cataracts,[79] kidney damage,[80] and adrenal gland dysfunction.[81]

NATURAL SWEETENERS

Natural and artificial sugar substitutes are available. However, artificial sweeteners have been linked to increased cancer risk.[82 83] Long-term use of artificial sweeteners has been linked to headaches, seizures, blindness, and cognitive and behavioral changes.[84]

Artificial sweeteners such as saccharin (Sugar Twin, Sweet 'N Low), aspartame (Equal, NutraSweet), sucralose (Splenda), acesulfame potassium (also known as acesulfame k—Sunett, Sweet One), neotame, and tagatose are linked to a number of health problems. Numerous studies show that frequent consumption of low-calorie artificial sweeteners causes weight gain and increases one's risk for metabolic syndrome, type 2 diabetes, and cardiovascular disease.[85]

The consumption of artificial sweeteners leads to increased body weight and obesity because it interferes with the normal functions of the body.[86] In one study, consumption of artificial sweeteners increased BMI and increased body fat percentage at a two-year follow-up.[87]

Even though low-calorie artificial sweeteners are currently approved for use, many people have reported that they believe their negative health symptoms were caused by these artificial sugar substitutes.[88]

Coconut palm sugar, stevia, and raw organic Manuka honey are the best natural sweeteners to use and even have some health benefits.

Coconut palm sugar is a very good sugar substitute. It is low on the GI (with a GI of 35), and rich in potassium, magnesium, zinc, iron, and B vitamins.

Stevia has been widely used for centuries in South America as well as in Japan. It has zero calories and has a GI of zero, which means it does not raise blood sugar levels. Unlike sugar, which has a negative effect on those with diabetes, stevia has been shown to have a positive effect on those with diabetes.[89] Studies have found that stevia improves insulin sensitivity,[90] promotes additional insulin production,[91] and helps reverse diabetes and metabolic syndrome.[92]

Ancient scriptures promote the use of honey. According to the Bible, "eat honey, for it is good" (NLT, Proverbs 24:13). The Quran calls honey a healing food (Saheeh International English Translation, Surah an-Nahl 16:68–69). In many ancient cultures, raw organic honey was used for medical purposes.[93]

The medicinal use of products made by honeybees is called apitherapy. The use of honey and propolis in the treatment and prevention of numerous diseases has been documented.[94] [95] Honey has demonstrated bactericidal activity against salmonella, Shigella, Escherichia coli, and H. pylori.[96]

Research demonstrates that propolis has the highest antioxidant power, followed by royal jelly and honey.[97] Propolis has antibacterial, antifungal, antiviral, antioxidative, antiparasitic, immunomodulating, anti-inflammatory, analgesic, hepatoprotective, and anti-carcinogenic effects.[98] Royal jelly has antitumor effects.[99 100 101]

The antibacterial activity in Manuka honey is much stronger than in other types of honey.[102] "UMF" stands for "Unique Manuka Factor" and is a property that gives Manuka honey its special healing quality. UMF Manuka honey with a rating of 16+ has the highest level of antibacterial activity. Manuka honey is best consumed raw, as heat destroys the nutrients in honey.[103]

RAW VS. COOKED

Cooking foods destroy their nutrients.[104] A German study found that high consumption of raw vegetables appears to decrease the risk of breast cancer. However, the increased intake of cooked vegetables did not contribute to the reduced risk of breast cancer, probably due to the loss of nutrients.[105]

If one chooses to cook vegetables, steaming seems to be the best cooking method for the retention of nutrients.[106]

The International Agency for Research on Cancer (IARC) has concluded that toxic compounds present in cooked meats may cause cancer.[107]

Researchers have found that high consumption of well-done, fried, or barbecued meats was associated with increased risks of colorectal cancer[108] and pancreatic cancer.[109] [200] Meat and fish should be eaten raw, like in sushi, or rare-cooked.

A healthy diet consists of a high percentage of raw, antioxidant-rich foods. A comprehensive study found that berries, fruits, vegetables, nuts, and dark chocolate have the highest antioxidant levels of all common foods.[201]

Chocolate has many documented health benefits, but because it's a calorie-dense food, it should be eaten in very small amounts. Overeating chocolate leads to weight gain. It's the cocoa that offers health benefits; therefore, choose only organic dark chocolate with a minimum cocoa content of 70 percent.[202]

FOOD PREPARATION

The best food preparation methods maintain the nutrients and health-promoting compounds in food. You want to avoid any cooking methods that devitalize food.

A study investigated common cooking methods—including steaming, microwaving, boiling, and stir-frying—and their effects on the nutrients and health-promoting compounds of broccoli. The results showed that all cooking treatments, except steaming, caused significant losses of valuable nutrients and healthful compounds.[203] [204] To retain nutritional values at maximum levels, vegetables are best prepared by steam cooking.

Certain cooking methods should be avoided due to their ability to increase cancer risk. Grilling and toasting produced substantial increases in cancer-causing compounds in bread. Microwave cooking produced elevated cancer-causing levels in some cheeses. Microwave cooking, frying, and broiling foods increase the risk of certain cancers and tumors.[205]

Microwaving is one of the worst cooking methods. The Nazis invented the first microwave-cooking device to provide food support to their troops during their invasion of the

Soviet Union in World War II. After the war, the Russians conducted thorough research on microwave ovens. Shocked by what they learned, the Russians banned microwave ovens in 1976, later lifting the ban during Perestroika. Russian investigators found that carcinogens were formed during the microwaving of nearly all foods tested. Microwaving fruits, vegetables, grains, milk, and meat caused the formation of cancer-causing substances. Microwaving led to decreased food value for all foods tested, with significant decreases in B-complex vitamins, vitamins C and E, essential minerals, and lipotropics (substances that prevent abnormal accumulation of fat).

Swiss food scientist Hans Hertel found that the consumption of microwaved food increased cholesterol levels, decreased numbers of white blood cells, and decreased numbers of red blood cells.

To prevent yourself from using a microwave oven and microwavable meals, prepare your meals ahead of time. Make soups and stews in bulk, then freeze them. An hour before mealtime, take one out and defrost it in a sink of water until it's thawed enough to slip into a pot, then reheat it on the stove.

SEAWEED

The soil on the earth has been depleted, but the sea is rich in minerals. Seaweeds are the richest source of minerals on the planet. They contain higher amounts of both macrominerals and trace elements than do land plants.[206]

The consumption of seaweed is an important factor contributing to the relatively low breast cancer rates reported in

Japan.[207] Research suggests that edible seaweeds prevent cancer.[208] Dulse (Palmaria palmata) is especially useful for preventing cancer.[209] Kelp has been shown to prevent breast tumors.[210] Wakame and kombu inhibited the growth of cancer cells significantly.[211] Mekabu (wakame root) may prevent breast cancer.[212]

Seaweed is an excellent source of iodine and helps people with hypothyroidism. However, make sure not to consume too much, as it can lead to iodine poisoning.

ORGANIC FOODS

Organic produce is nutritionally superior to conventional produce. Organic food is produced without antibiotics, artificial ingredients, chemical preservatives, genetic engineering, irradiation, synthetic fertilizers, synthetic hormones, and pesticides.

According to the Environmental Protection Agency, fungicides, herbicides, and insecticides can be carcinogenic. Pesticides can be neurotoxins, endocrine disruptors, and immune system suppressors. When you are not eating food that is 100 percent organic, you are consuming food that contains poisonous chemicals.[213] Pesticides, insecticides, herbicides, and fungicides are found in food that is not organic and has been shown to cause cancer.[214]

Researchers found that antioxidant levels were higher in those consuming a Mediterranean diet consisting of organic food versus one consisting of conventional food.[215] Organic foods contain higher concentrations of antioxidants.[216] Organic foods contain significantly more nutrients with lower amounts of some heavy metals as compared to conventional foods.[217][218]

The best possible thing to do is to grow your own organic fruits and vegetables. Watering the soil with ozonated water and treating it with volcanic or humic shale and seawater will ensure produce that is rich in nutrients. If you can't grow your own food, buy biodynamic organic produce whenever you can.

Choose the freshest organic produce. If you are unable to purchase super-fresh organic produce, buy frozen organic fruits and vegetables. Freezing has little effect on the nutrient content of food.

It is especially essential to buy organic white potatoes, sweet potatoes, ginger, garlic, and onions because if they are not organic, they have been treated with sprout inhibitors that have dangerous DNA-damaging effects causing cancer.[219][220][221][222]

CALCIUM AND MILK

Many people do not digest and assimilate cow's milk properly, typically because of lactose and casein. Many people do much better on milk from other animals, such as sheep or goats.[223] Cow's milk is a common cause of digestive problems, allergies, and excess mucous, but goat's and sheep's milk are not. Both sheep's and goat's milk have a higher nutritional value and are better digested than is cow's milk.[224]

Goat's and sheep's milk are not only more easily digested and nutritious, but also less toxic. Most cows are pumped full of synthetic hormones and antibiotics, but goats and sheep are typically not treated with these substances.

Whole goat's milk contains vitamins A and D, as well as B vitamins and the minerals calcium, magnesium, phosphorous, and potassium.

Sheep's milk is commonly consumed in the Mediterranean. Greek feta cheese and Italian ricotta cheese are typically made from sheep's milk. Many people consider sheep's milk better-tasting than cow's milk and goat's milk because it has a rich, creamy, sweet taste. Whole sheep's milk is richer in protein and calcium than either cow's or goat's milk. It contains higher levels of conjugated linoleic acid that promote fat loss. It also contains phosphorous, magnesium, potassium, zinc, vitamin A, and B vitamins.

In addition to sheep's milk and goat's milk, more and more people are looking for other good alternatives to cow's milk due to allergies and intolerance. Certain animals produce milk that has healing properties, and this milk is used as a medicine in some cultures.

Camel's milk reportedly has powerful healing properties. It can heal gut problems, autoimmune conditions, autism, and diabetes.[225] [226] Those with severe food allergies are in many cases able to consume camel's milk, and astonishingly, fully recover from their allergies to all foods.[227]

Bedouin parents give their children camel's milk for a couple weeks during their childhoods, as they know that it builds a strong immune system for life.

Camels are unlike any other mammal. They can survive in incredibly harsh climates, and are able to live without water for 30 days at a time while still producing high-quality milk. The healing power of camel's milk likely stems from the animal's unique, hardy build and strong survival ability.

Camel's milk has incredible antibacterial and antiviral properties because it contains immunoglobulins and protective proteins.[228] Camel's milk helps treat liver problems and boosts immunity.[229]

Mare's milk, also called horse milk, can overcome inflammatory and various skin disorders such as dermatitis.[230] Fermented mare's milk was found to have a high antioxidant capacity, and research has shown that it has a protective property against the toxic effects of mercury in the body.[231] Mare's milk is considered by some to be closer in composition to human milk than any other mammal's milk.

Raw donkey's milk was used as a cure for a variety of illnesses. The Greek physician Hippocrates recommended it to treat liver problems, fevers, infectious diseases, poisoning, joint pain, and nosebleeds. Donkey's milk contains antibacterial, anti-inflammatory, and anti-allergen properties reported to heal psoriasis, eczema, asthma, and bronchitis.[232][233]

Wild elk's milk, also known as moose milk, is used as a treatment for duodenal and gastric ulcers. The healing properties of wild elk could be due to the elks' diet. In the wild, they eat grasses, shrubs, and approximately 350 species of forest plants, many of which have medicinal value. Elk's milk also has antibacterial effects.

Buffalo's milk is a rich source of calcium, magnesium, potassium, and phosphorus. Buffalo's milk is thick and creamy, and many prefer its taste over that of cow's milk.

Tibetan nomads have lived since ancient times in the harsh environment of the Qinghai-Tibetan Plateau, with average altitudes of over 4,000 meters. They have been able to live healthy lives and reproduce despite being under the extreme stress of a high-altitude environment that includes cold, hypoxia, and strong ultraviolet radiation. They have been able to thrive on a simple diet consisting mainly of yak's milk and its products. The Tibetan nomads' diet is devoid of vegetables and fruits for most of the year. Yak's milk is a complete food consisting of high levels of antioxidant vitamins, enzymes, probiotics, amino acids, and fatty acids.[234]

Milk is best consumed raw and unpasteurized, as it contains the most nutrients and healing properties in this form. Raw, organic milk from grass-fed animals was used as a medicine in the 1920s. Raw milk was used to treat—and frequently cure—some serious chronic diseases.[235]

The Mayo Foundation used a diet of raw milk as a remedy for heart failure, diabetes, kidney disease, chronic fatigue, and obesity. In Germany, raw milk therapy is used by many hospitals.[236] Raw milk prevents tooth decay, even in children who eat a lot of sugar.[237]

Raw milk is superior to pasteurized milk because heating milk destroys many nutrients.[238] Raw milk can be purchased from a farmer or a farmer's market. Use an Internet search engine to find local, raw, grass-fed milk and fermented milk products. You can also visit www.realmilk.com to find high-quality milk in your area.

If you cannot gain access to raw, grass-fed milk, you will be better off to completely remove fresh milk from your diet and consume only organic, grass-fed fermented milk products.

Research demonstrated an association between pasteurized milk consumption and the development of diseases such as type 2 diabetes. In contrast, fermented milk products exhibit an inverse correlation.[239]

Raw milk is generally not associated with the health problems linked to pasteurized milk, and even people who are allergic to pasteurized milk can typically tolerate and even thrive on raw milk. Grass-fed dairy has a high amount of conjugated linoleic acid (CLA). CLA raises your metabolic rate, allowing you to burn fat.

Those with an intolerance or allergic reaction to fresh milk are able to consume ghee, clarified butter, buttermilk, cultured cream, kefir, full-fat yogurt, clabber, and other fermented milk products. Fermented milk products often contain probiotics, which promote gut health. Greek yogurt is a good option, as it has twice as much protein as regular yogurt.

Those who would rather not consume milk can get their calcium from arame, kombu, or sesame seeds. Arame and kombu are extremely high in calcium. Arame contains 1,170 milligrams per 100 grams, kombu contains 800 milligrams per 100 grams, and sesame seeds contain 630 milligrams per 100 grams. Milk (two percent) has only 297 milligrams per cup.

ORGANIC GRASS-FED MEAT

If an animal isn't fed nutritious food, it won't become nutritious food. Feeding an animal junk turns it into junk food. Ruminant animals are meant to eat grass.

To attain the optimum weight gain in a minimum amount of time, animals used for food (cows, pigs, chickens, sheep) are administered growth-stimulating hormones and feed additives. They are fed corn, soybean, sorghum, and other grains. This grain feed is high in insecticides. When consumed by the animals, the pesticides accumulate in their bodies. The pesticides are then passed along to the consumer. Beef ranks second only to tomatoes as the food posing the greatest cancer risk due to pesticide contamination, according to the National Research Council of the National Academy of Sciences.

Some feedlot operators give their animals cardboard, newspaper, candy, sawdust, chicken feces, ground-up rock, sewage, and garbage. They do this to reduce costs and fatten animals more quickly, with a lack of regard for the health effects on consumers. Some factory farms scrape up the manure from chicken houses and pigpens and add it directly to cattle feed. Food and Drug Administration (FDA) officials say that it's not uncommon for some feedlot operators to mix industrial sewage and oils into the feed.

Conventionally raised meat is higher in calories and less nutritious. Grass-fed meat is lower in calories. It also contains more omega-3 fats, more vitamins A and E, and up to seven times the beta-carotene compared to conventionally raised meat. "If you eat a typical amount of beef per year, which in the United States is about 67 pounds, switching to grass-fed beef will save you 16,642 calories a year," states Jo Robinson in *Pasture Perfect*, a book about the benefits of pasture-raised meat.

The longer an animal is fed grains, the lower the nutrient content of the meat. The omega-3 quantity of grain-fed meat is so low it doesn't qualify as a good dietary source. Grass-fed meat has enough omega-3 to be considered a good source of omega-3 fatty acids.[240]

Omega-3 fatty acids prevent sudden cardiac death. They lower blood pressure and heart rate, improve blood vessel function, lower triglycerides, and reduce inflammation.[241] Grass-fed beef, walnuts, flaxseed, sardines, and salmon are good sources of omega-3 fatty acids.

Meat and dairy products from grass-fed meat are the richest sources of conjugated linoleic acid (CLA). CLA is a naturally occurring trans-fatty acid that improves brain function, promotes weight loss, and reduces the risk of cancer. When animals are raised on grass, their products contain three to five times more CLA than do meat from animals fed grain.[242]

Heterocyclic amines (HCAs) and polycyclic aromatic hydrocarbons (PAHs) are chemicals formed when meat is cooked using high temperatures (above 300° F) or for a long time, such as when pan frying, barbecuing, smoking, charring, or grilling directly over an open flame. HCAs and PAHs have been found to cause changes in DNA that may increase the risk of cancer.[243] [244] Researchers found that frequent consumption of well-done, fried, or barbecued meat was associated with increased risks of colorectal[245] pancreatic,[246] [247] and prostate cancer.[248] [249] Meat should be eaten rare-cooked or braised in water or stock.

Processed meats such as sausage, luncheon meats, pastrami, salami, hot dogs, and bacon contain preservatives that increase cancer risk.[250] Lacto-fermentation or salt curing are old-fashioned and better ways to preserve meat.

Vary the types of meat you eat. Most people consume only chicken, beef, and pork. Try wild game meats such as goat, bison, deer, antelope, elk, kangaroo, and game birds such as partridge, quail, duck, goose, and pheasant.

ORGANIC FREE-RANGE EGGS

Eggs, especially the yolk, contain all the essential amino acids and essential fatty acids and are a good source of selenium, phosphorus, vitamin A, vitamin B2, vitamin B5, vitamin B6, folic acid, vitamin B12, vitamins E and D, choline, lutein, and zeaxanthin.

A chicken's diet has an effect on the nutritional quality of its eggs. Eggs from free-range chickens are more nutritious than conventional eggs. They are higher in vitamins A and E, and in omega-3.[251] Omega-3 eggs had 5 to 10 times as much omega-3 as did conventional eggs.[252]

Any pesticides and herbicides present in the diet of chickens can end up in their eggs. Organic eggs do not contain antibiotics or hormones, but the chickens may not have had access to the outdoors.

Eggs are nutritious, high-protein, high-satiety foods. They are ideal for breakfast. Research shows that eating eggs for breakfast promotes weight loss. Several meta-analyses strongly suggest that daily egg consumption does not adversely affect plasma lipoproteins with regard to the risk of coronary heart disease or stroke.[253]

Some people eat only the egg whites for their protein content. However, it's the egg yolks that are the most nutritious part of the egg; the egg white has very few vitamins and minerals. Egg yolks contain fat-soluble vitamins A, D, E, and K as well as all the carotenoids, lutein, and zeaxanthin found in an egg. They also contain calcium, iron, phosphorus, zinc, thiamin, folate, vitamin B6, and vitamin B12.

Organic egg yolks can be eaten raw or added to a smoothie, while raw egg whites should not be eaten raw, as they contain several protease inhibitors and anti-nutrients that interfere with the digestion of proteins and can result in a biotin deficiency.

Raw eggs carry the risk of salmonella contamination, although the risk of infection from raw or undercooked eggs is minimal when the eggs are organic and free-range and washed before consumption.

Most people eat only chicken's eggs. However, eggs from certain other birds are even more nutritious. If you can find them, purchase eggs from ducks, geese, quail, turkeys, ostriches, pheasants, or emus. Most people who are allergic to chicken eggs can eat other types of bird eggs without allergic reactions. The best places to find different types of eggs are farmers' markets, gourmet food stores, and higher-end grocery stores like Whole Foods Market (www.wholefoodsmarket.com).

Duck eggs have higher levels of nutrients than do chicken eggs and stay fresher longer because of their thicker shells. Ducks eggs have higher levels of vitamin D, vitamin A, vitamin E, vitamin K2, and omega-3 fatty acids.

Eggs are fairly high in cholesterol, but it's a myth that cholesterol has a negative effect on cholesterol levels in people with normal cholesterol metabolism. To put things in perspective, one egg contains the same amount of saturated fat as a small tablespoon of olive oil.

Cooking destroys some of the heat-sensitive nutrients, like certain B vitamins. The longer eggs are cooked, the more nutrients are lost. The best cooking methods—like sunny side up or poached—leave the egg yolk intact and soft.

OMEGA-3-RICH FISH

Fish are a good source of protein; most varieties contain around 20 grams of protein per three-ounce serving. Fish is also a good source of vitamin B12, iron, vitamins A and D, and omega-3 fatty acids. Certain varieties of fish are higher in omega-3 than others. Salmon, mackerel, halibut, herring, lake trout and sardines are the fish with the highest omega-3 fatty acid content.

Fish and shellfish have been shown to contain varying amounts of heavy metals, particularly mercury and fat-soluble pollutants from water pollution. They often concentrate mercury in their bodies in the form of methylmercury, a highly toxic organic compound of mercury. Methylmercury is not soluble and thus is not excreted from the body.[254]

Wild fish generally have lower levels of toxins than farmed fish. Coastal and farmed salmon may have higher levels. The Environmental Working Group (EWG) has analyzed research and found that farmed salmon contains 16 times more polychlorinated biphenyl (PCBs) than do wild salmon. PCBs are very toxic cancer-causing chemicals that accumulate in human tissues and organs over time and are difficult to eliminate from the body even with cleansing and detoxing regimens.

Species of fish that are long-lived and high on the food chain, such as marlins, tuna, sharks, swordfish, king mackerel, tilefish, and northern pike, contain high concentrations of mercury. Swordfish and bluefin tuna have been found to contain the highest concentrations of mercury of all fish species.[255] Fish and shellfish have also been found to possess lead and cadmium.[256]

Those who would like to reap the health benefits of fish can consume wild-caught Alaskan salmon instead of Atlantic or Norwegian salmon. A study found that wild Alaskan salmon had the lowest level of contaminants as compared to Atlantic salmon and organically farmed Norwegian salmon.[257] Studies show that farmed salmon has consistently higher levels of contaminants than does wild salmon.[258][259][260]

A study that analyzed mercury levels in humans from 32 locations in 13 countries found that mercury levels were highest in the group that ate fish once or more per day.[261]

A study concluded that the benefits of fish intake exceed the potential risks. Moderate consumption of fish, especially species higher in omega-3, reduces the risk of coronary death by 36 percent and total mortality by 17 percent.[262]

A study analyzed the foods that pose the greatest cancer risk due to certain contaminants (arsenic, chlordane, dichlorodiphenyltrichloroethane (DDT), dieldrin, dioxins, and PCBs). Shellfish and fish (saltwater and freshwater) are significant contributors to the total exposures for some contaminants (arsenic and PCBs in shellfish; arsenic, chlordane, dieldrin, dioxin, and PCBs in fish). After fish, the largest contributors to chemical exposure are other meat and animal products, including beef, chicken, pork, and milk.[263] Farmed fish and crude fish oil contain brominated flame-retardants (BFRs).[264]

You want to eat fish and shellfish in moderation and get most of your protein needs from sources low in contaminants such as free-range eggs and wild game. When selecting fish, consume only wild-caught, cold-water fish rather than farmed fish.

ORGANIC UNROASTED NUTS

Many people avoid eating nuts because they are high in fat and calories. However, numerous epidemiological and clinical studies show that frequent consumption of nuts is not associated with weight gain because they are very satiating, boost metabolism, have a thermogenic effect, and have low metabolizable energy (meaning that you don't absorb all of the calories).

Clinical trials have shown that people do not gain weight when they include various types of nuts in their diets.[265] [266] "Nuts suppress hunger as well as the desire to eat," explains Dr. Richard Mattes, MPH, PhD, RD. He recommends a maximum of 40 grams per day of unsalted nuts, such as almonds, walnuts, and Brazil nuts.

Nuts are rich sources of nutrients such as vitamin E, magnesium, selenium, folate, essential fatty acids, fiber, protein, and phytochemicals. They offer numerous health benefits, including a reduced risk of cardiovascular disease and diabetes.[267]

When you need a dessert or treat, eat a handful of your favorite nuts. Nuts raise your basal metabolic rate, meaning they raise the rate at which you burn calories. In one study, two weeks of overeating candy led to higher LDL cholesterol, increased insulin levels, and weight gain. Overeating nuts led to an increased basal metabolic rate and did not cause the same negative metabolic effects as eating candy did.[268]

Nuts are a very good addition to your breakfast because they promote fullness, reduce appetite, and prevent spikes in blood sugar throughout the morning and even after the next meal of the day.[269]

Nuts are an indispensable part of a healthy diet and should be in everyone's regimen. A balanced, healthy diet like the Mediterranean diet is high in nuts, seeds, vegetables, fruits, pulses, whole grains, meat, and dairy products. The Mediterranean diet and frequent consumption of nuts prevent life-threatening diseases such as coronary heart disease.[270][271]

Raw, organic, unroasted, unsalted nuts to incorporate in your diet include almonds, walnuts, Brazil nuts, cashews, hazelnuts, macadamia nuts, pecans, pine nuts, and pistachios.

WHOLE GRAINS AND PULSES

Whole grains have high concentrations of essential nutrients, antioxidants, and fiber. Studies have found that consumption of whole grains promotes weight loss.[272] The dietary fiber found in whole grains helps promote a feeling of satiety, which reduces the amount of food eaten. Consumption of whole grains lowers BMI, WHR, total cholesterol, and LDL cholesterol.[273]

There is an overwhelming amount of scientific evidence showing the health benefits offered by the consumption of whole grains.[274] Whole grains contain a wide range of phytochemicals with numerous health benefits.[275]

Diets high in whole grains are associated with a 20 to 30 percent reduction in the risk of type-2 diabetes.[278] The disease protection offered by the consumption of whole grains far exceeds the benefits from isolated nutrients and phytochemicals found in nutritional supplements.[279]

Pulses (beans, peas, lentils) are a source of protein and fiber as well as a significant source of vitamins and minerals such as iron, zinc, folate, and magnesium. Pulses are high in fiber and have a low GI. They are very beneficial to people with diabetes because they help maintain a balanced blood sugar level. Pulses have anti-cancer effects, as they contain phytochemicals, saponins, and tannins.[280]

Scientific evidence indicates that whole grains play an important role in lowering the risk of chronic diseases such as coronary heart disease, diabetes, and various types of cancer, and also contribute to body weight management and gastrointestinal health.[281]

Dr. Price discovered that the healthiest cultures include whole grains and pulses in their diets. However, they usually soak or ferment their grains and pulses before eating them to neutralize phytates and enzyme inhibitors. Fermented or soaked grains are predigested, making them easy to digest with all nutrients more readily available.

Grains contain phytic acid, which combines with iron, calcium, magnesium, copper, and zinc in the intestinal tract, blocking their absorption.[282]

Many people who are allergic to certain grains, beans, or legumes are able to eat them without a problem if they are properly prepared. Soak grains and pulses for seven hours or more before cooking, sprouting, or sour leavening.

To soak grains or pulses, put them in a bowl, cover them with enough water, and add a tablespoon of either yogurt, raw apple cider vinegar, lemon juice, or kefir. Allow them to sit at room temperature for at least seven hours. Drain and rinse before cooking them with fresh water.

Grains you want to stay away from include white rice, refined white flour, granola, and—if you have celiac disease or a gluten sensitivity—grains containing gluten.

Refined carbohydrates such as white rice and white flour may contribute to type 2 diabetes and cardiovascular disease. Modern Asian Indians (people from India, Pakistan, and Bangladesh) typically include a lot of white rice and refined white flour in their diet, which may contribute to the remarkably high prevalence of type 2 diabetes and cardiovascular disease in this population.[283]

Granola which is labeled a "healthy cereal" is made from grains subjected only to dry heat, making it extremely indigestible. Granola, like all processed breakfast cereals, is not healthy as some people think.

Hot and cold breakfast porridge made from properly prepared, low GI, nutritious whole grains such as amaranth, quinoa, and teff are good substitutes for commercial breakfast cereals and granola.

The best whole grains are ancient grains prized for their high nutritional content, such as quinoa, amaranth, barley, millet, couscous, buckwheat, teff, bulgur, farro, kamut, and spelt. Most ancient grains are gluten-free, high in fiber, and high in essential nutrients. They reduce cholesterol levels and offer a number of other health benefits. Many ancient grains can be used in recipes for bread, pancakes, crepes, waffles, muffins, and cookies, and can be eaten as hot breakfast cereals. Ancient whole grains can be found in health food stores.

Quinoa is a complete protein source, containing all the essential amino acids. Quinoa is about 14 percent protein, a high level for a plant-based food. The red and yellow varieties of quinoa may have a slightly higher protein content than does white quinoa. Quinoa contains dietary fiber, phosphorus, magnesium, and iron. Quinoa is also gluten free.

Amaranth is about 14 percent protein. Researchers concluded that the protein in amaranth "is among the highest in nutritive quality of vegetable origin and close to those of animal origin products."[284] Amaranth is gluten-free and a good source of vitamins A, B6, K, and C, as well as folate and riboflavin. Amaranth is an excellent source of manganese, iron, calcium, copper, magnesium, phosphorus, and potassium.

Buckwheat doesn't contain gluten, making it an ideal dietary option for those who are gluten sensitive or who have celiac disease. Buckwheat contains the eight essential amino acids and is rich in B vitamins as well as phosphorus, magnesium, iron, folate, zinc, copper, and manganese. Buckwheat is high in fiber. A single cup of cooked buckwheat groats contains over four grams of dietary fiber.

Teff is gluten-free and rich in vitamins and minerals such as manganese, potassium, phosphorus, magnesium, calcium, iron, vitamin C, niacin, vitamin A, and thiamin. One serving of teff (a quarter cup) offers seven grams of protein and four grams of fiber. When cooked on a stovetop with water, it creates a creamy product similar to cream of wheat, making it a good option for a hot breakfast cereal.

Pearled barley is an excellent source of vitamins B1, B2, B3, B6, and B9. Pearled barley has the lowest GI of all the common grains, including wheat, rye, and oats. The GI of boiled pearled barley is 35, so it is considered a low-glycemic food and a good choice for diabetics.

Brown rice and wild rice are good sources of the B vitamins, vitamin E, and the minerals potassium, phosphorus, calcium, magnesium, and manganese. Brown and wild rice contain both the germ and the bran of the grain and are considered healthier than white rice because they contain more nutrients and fiber. In contrast, white rice has the germ and bran of the grain polished away and therefore contains fewer nutrients and less fiber.

Rice has been a staple food for many generations—and for good reason. It is easy to digest and highly nutritious. In the oldest known book of Chinese medicine, *Classic of Internal Medicine*, the first remedy for disease treatment is a 10-day period during which the patient eats only rice.

Different varieties of rice have different GI indices depending on their fiber content and amylose content. Worldwide, there are more than 40,000 varieties of rice. Many varieties, especially white rice, are classified as high GI foods. Look for rice with high fiber and high amylose content, which means the rice will be low on the GI. Doongara rice has a higher amylose content and is low on the GI.[285 286 287]

Long-grain brown rice and basmati rice are also low on the GI.[288 289] Of all varieties of rice, Koshihikari rice, and Bangladeshi rice are the lowest on the GI.[290]

Millet is gluten-free whole grain that can be consumed by people with celiac disease or those with allergies or intolerance to gluten. It is rich in B vitamins, especially niacin, B6, and folic acid, as well as the minerals calcium, iron, potassium, magnesium, and zinc. Millet has a high GI and therefore should be consumed in small amounts and eaten only in combination with protein and healthy fats. Millet can be made into a delicious hot breakfast. A porridge can be made with goat's or sheep's milk, nuts, seeds, cinnamon, flaxseed, and stevia or raw Manuka honey added at the end of the cooking process. Millet can also be boiled in water with apples added during the boiling process and raw honey, cinnamon, and nuts or seeds added during the cooling process.

Fonio is a kind of millet—a cross between couscous and quinoa in both appearance and texture. It has been cultivated in West Africa for thousands of years and is used in salads, stews, and porridges, as well as ground into flour. It is gluten-free and a great alternative for gluten-intolerant people. Fonio is rich in B vitamins, magnesium, zinc, manganese, and amino acids, particularly in the amino acids methionine and cysteine.

Couscous is made from semolina, a form of wheat. People with celiac disease or those who have gluten intolerance will generally not be able to eat couscous. Couscous is rich in B vitamins and the minerals calcium, phosphorus, selenium, potassium, and magnesium. A one-cup serving of cooked couscous provides six grams of protein and two grams of dietary fiber. Couscous is a staple food in Africa, Europe, the Middle East, India, and many other parts of the world. It can be added to a soup or to meat and vegetable dishes, or consumed as a dessert when dates, sesame, and honey are added to it.

Bulgur is made from the groats of several different wheat species, typically durum wheat. Bulgur has been a staple of the traditional Mediterranean diet for thousands of years. People with celiac disease or those who have gluten intolerance will not be able to eat bulgur. It has a low GI of 48. It is high in fiber and protein, and low in calories. It is rich in B vitamins, iron, phosphorous, and manganese.

Farro has significantly less gluten than wheat does. Farro is the oldest cultivated grain in the world. In ancient Rome, farro was a staple food of the Roman legions. It is common in many traditional Mediterranean dishes. In Italy, the most common way to eat farro is by adding it to soup. It can also be added to salads and made into pasta and bread. A half cup contains four grams of fiber and four grams of protein.

Freekeh is made from young wheat (typically durum) that is harvested while still green. It has been a staple of Middle Eastern diets for centuries. It's not a gluten-free grain, but some people with gluten intolerance are able to consume it. Freekeh is low on the GI and suitable for those with diabetes. It is a high-fiber, high-protein grain that is more nutrient-rich than many other grains. It is high in iron, calcium, zinc, selenium, potassium, and magnesium.

Some people who are allergic to wheat report better results when they use ancient varieties of wheat, like kamut or spelt. You can substitute kamut flour or spelt flour in any recipe calling for wheat flour, such as pasta, bread, waffles, crepes, pancakes, muffins, cakes, cookies, crackers, or baked goods. Spelt has higher amounts of protein, B vitamins, potassium, and iron than do other varieties of wheat. Kamut contains calcium, iron, magnesium, phosphorus, potassium, and zinc.

LONG-FERMENTED BREAD

Gluten sensitivity is so common that many nutritionists recommend avoiding the consumption of grains and bread. Dr. Price studied several societies that enjoyed perfect health and were completely free from disease. He found that they consumed grains and bread prepared the old-fashioned way.

Some people with celiac disease or gluten sensitivity are able to eat bread prepared with long fermentation. The long, slow fermentation process of over 18 to 25 hours digests and breaks down the gluten and also neutralizes enzyme inhibitors that interfere with digestion and phytic acid that blocks nutrient absorption. Fermentation also lowers the GI of bread. Bread prepared in this old-fashioned way is highly nutritious, providing many nutrients in a form that is delicious and very easy to digest.

"Most of the plastic-wrap bread you find at grocery stores is made very quickly with yeast—it goes from flour to plastic-wrap in three hours or less," says Stephen Jones, a wheat breeder. Gluten proteins don't have time to break down, and it is very hard to digest.

In the long, slow fermentation process that produces sourdough bread, nutrients such as iron, zinc, and magnesium, as well as antioxidants, folic acid, and other B vitamins, are made available. Sourdough bread produces a lower surge in blood sugar than any other bread.[291]

A study found that people with celiac disease who ate sourdough bread for 60 days had no clinical complaints. Their biopsies showed no changes in their intestinal linings. The researchers concluded that sourdough bread is safe to consume for the majority of people with celiac disease.[292]

You can make your own bread or buy traditional long-fermented bread from artisan bakers who make bread the old-fashioned way. Be sure to buy "whole-milled" whole wheat flour. This kind of flour has been milled from its intact state.

You want to completely avoid bread and baked goods made from white flour and whole wheat flour that has not been "whole-milled." Factory bread producers separate the endosperm from the more nutritious bran and germ. Although they are added back to whole wheat flour, craft bakers speculate that the germ, which goes rancid when removed from the endosperm, is either not added back or is "denatured." Therefore, purchase only bread and baked goods made with "whole-milled" whole wheat flour.

White flour has the germ and bran removed (along with 80 percent of the fiber and most of the nutrients). White flours are usually fortified, but the flour is still missing many healthy compounds, such as antioxidants and phytonutrients. White flour and many varieties of whole wheat bread are higher than sugar on the GI, typically around 71. Table sugar (sucrose) is 58 on the GI.

LACTO-FERMENTED FOODS

For centuries, cultures around the world have been eating traditional fermented foods and beverages for their benefits, which include increased longevity and improved digestive health.

Fermented foods and beverages are produced or preserved by the action of microorganisms. This lacto-fermentation process preserves the food and creates beneficial enzymes, B vitamins, omega-3 fatty acids, and various strains of probiotics.

The WHO has defined probiotics as "live organisms which when administered in adequate amounts confer a health benefit on the host."

The gastrointestinal tract is colonized by about 10 trillion microbes of many different species, both good and bad. Probiotics are often called "good" or "beneficial" bacteria because they help keep your gut healthy. When there are more "bad" bacteria, health problems can develop. Probiotics lower the amount of "bad" bacteria in the gut.

Research has discovered that probiotics provide many health benefits for humans when ingested. They are beneficial for both disease prevention and treatment.[293] They improve immune health and help treat diseases, such as allergies, eczema, viral infections, urogenital infections, cystic fibrosis, and various cancers.[294] [295] They prevent and treat gastrointestinal infections, irritable bowel syndrome (IBS), inflammatory bowel disease (IBD), and food allergies.[296] [297] They improve digestive health and help you absorb more of the nutrients in the foods you eat, reducing such unpleasant symptoms as bloating.[298]

There are many types of fermented foods and beverages such as sauerkraut, kimchi, kefir, fermented milk, kombucha, brem, chass, amasi, kvass, and ayran, to name just a few.

BONE BROTH

Bone broths made from beef, chicken, fish, and lamb bones have been staples of the traditional diets of every culture for thousands of years. "Good broth will resurrect the dead," says a South American proverb; though this might be an embellishment, bone broth is very beneficial.

Organic homemade bone broth contains high amounts of essential nutrients that play an important role in strong, healthy bones. It also improves digestion, fights infections, and reduces joint pain and inflammation. Practitioners of Chinese medicine have used bone broth to support the digestive system, as a blood builder, and to strengthen the kidneys.

Make your own bone broth or buy it from someone who makes it the authentic way instead of getting it from a restaurant or the store. Sally Fallon Morell, president of the Weston A. Price Foundation, explains that many store-bought broths aren't beneficial. These store-bought artificial broths are made using lab-produced meat flavors found in bouillon cubes and soup mixes. They also commonly add MSG. Even broth soup available at most restaurants are typically made with a prepackaged powdered soup base.

To make bone broth, select bone, marrow, feet (chicken feet) or tails (ox tail) from grass-fed animals free of antibiotics and hormones. Boil and then simmer the bones over a period of several hours. Simmering causes the bones and ligaments to release healthy compounds like gelatin, proline, and glycine. Glycine and proline are two key components of connective tissue. Glycine helps regulate blood sugar levels by controlling gluconeogenesis. In the brain, glycine inhibits excitatory neurotransmitters, producing a calming effect and helping you sleep better. Therefore, bone broth is very beneficial to drink before going to sleep or as a "souper."

CIDER AND RICE VINEGAR

For over 2,000 years, people have used vinegar to preserve and flavor food, disinfect wounds, and treat various ailments, from stomachaches to diabetes.

The most beneficial types of vinegar are rice vinegar and apple cider vinegar. Research has found that apple cider vinegar can help reduce weight.[299] "It may have some benefits in terms of weight loss and weight management," says Debbie Davis, a registered dietitian.

Apple cider vinegar has been found to lower serum cholesterol levels and protect the body against free radicals.[300] It also appears to help with diabetes and blood sugar control. Carol Johnston, PhD, has been studying apple cider vinegar for over 10 years and believes that its effect on blood sugar levels is similar to that of certain medications. "Apple cider vinegar's anti-glycemic effect is very well documented," says Johnston. Vinegar blocks some of the digestion of starch. "It doesn't block the starch 100 percent, but it definitely prevents at least some of that starch from being digested and raising your blood sugar," explains Johnston.

There is evidence that vinegar increases short-term satiety. Numerous studies found that blood sugar was better regulated after a meal that included vinegar.[301] Consuming vinegar with a meal leads to greater cell sensitivity to insulin and reduced production of glucose in the liver. Increased sensitivity to insulin leads to lower blood sugar after a meal. "Acetate (from vinegar) alters your metabolism to encourage fat breakdown rather than fat storage," explains Davis.

In North African cultures, women have used apple cider vinegar to achieve weight loss for generations. Bodybuilders are also known to use apple cider vinegar for weight reduction. However, you want to be careful about drinking apple cider vinegar because it causes erosive tooth wear.[302] It's so acidic that it will harm your tooth enamel and your esophagus. Dilute one to two tablespoons in a big glass of water and sip it along with your meals one or two times a day. You can also use apple cider vinegar in salads or add it to meals.

A study found that acetic acid killed cancer cells—specifically stomach cancer—and may also work to treat other types of cancer. "Acetic acid is a powerful anticancer agent," wrote Susumu Okabe, lead author of the study.[303]

Vinegar offers antioxidant protection and reduces cancer risk. Japanese rice vinegar (Kurosu) is particularly rich in the phenolic compounds that reduce cancer risk and has significantly greater antioxidant activity than other vinegar extracts, including wine and apple cider vinegar.[304 305]

You can make your own salad dressing with vinegar instead of buying commercially prepared salad dressings that contain sugar and preservatives. To make homemade salad dressing, combine rice vinegar or apple cider vinegar, flaxseed oil, lemon juice, Celtic sea salt, pepper, and chopped fresh herbs such as basil and thyme. You can also add raw Manuka honey for a sweet-flavored salad dressing.

COLD-PRESSED FLAXSEED OIL

Flaxseed has many health benefits. It is a powerful anti-inflammatory and immunomodulatory. It is an excellent source of omega-3 in the form of alpha-linolenic acid (ALA), not to be confused with alpha lipoic acid (ALA).

Alpha-linolenic acid is used for preventing and treating diseases of the heart and blood vessels. It is also used to treat rheumatoid arthritis (RA), multiple sclerosis (MS), lupus, diabetes, renal disease, ulcerative colitis, Crohn's disease, chronic obstructive pulmonary disease (COPD), migraine headaches, skin cancers, depression, and allergic and inflammatory conditions such as psoriasis and eczema.[306 307 308]

There is sufficient scientific evidence that alpha-linolenic acid from flaxseed is effective at preventing heart attacks, lowering high blood pressure, lowering cholesterol, and reversing hardening of the blood vessels (atherosclerosis).

The fiber found in flaxseed increases satiety and feelings of fullness.[309] Flaxseed fiber in beverage form and flaxseed capsules suppress the appetite, produce feelings of satiety, and reduce the intake of food.[310] A clinical study found that flaxseed promotes weight loss and decreases risk factors related to cardiovascular disease.[311] It reduces total and LDL cholesterol levels and liver disease risk factors.[312][313] A study found that flaxseed oil helps treat obesity-related inflammation and obesity-induced insulin resistance.[314] It decreased fasting blood sugar and cholesterol in type 2 diabetics.[315]

Flaxseed can be bought in a health food store, then ground into a powder at home with a flaxseed grinder and added to smoothies or drinks.

Flaxseed oil is very unstable and, when exposed to heat, light, or oxygen, becomes rancid much faster than do most other oils. Rancid oils contain free radicals that cause disease and that should be strictly avoided. Thus, don't purchase flaxseed oil unless it is very high quality, unrefined, cold-pressed, and stored in a dark, light-blocking bottle that is kept refrigerated at all times. The same rancidity issues are true for all other oils that are high in omega-3.

EXTRA VIRGIN COCONUT OIL

Coconuts are commonly consumed in Malaysia, Thailand, and the Philippines, and their oils are used as a complementary medicine. Clinical studies have shown that consumption of medium-chain saturated fatty acids (MCTs) such as coconut oil promotes weight loss and reduces fat around the stomach.[316][317]

Coconut oil has an abundance of lauric acid, which has many health benefits. In the body, lauric acid is converted into monolaurin, which exhibits antiviral, antimicrobial, antiprotozoal, and antifungal properties. It can be used to fight viruses, bacterial infections, and fungal infections. Researchers have found that lauric acid helps fights HIV/AIDS because of its strong antiviral properties.[318]

The consumption of coconut oil reduces total cholesterol and LDL levels.[319] It has also been found to help treat chronic stress and depression. A high-quality virgin coconut oil can rival antidepressant drugs without the dangerous side effects.[320]

Bruce Fife, a certified nutritionist, naturopathic physician, and author of *The Coconut Oil Miracle*, recommends that the average person consumes about three tablespoons of organic, extra virgin coconut oil per day. This amount will not only provide protection against bacteria and viruses but also increase metabolism. If you prefer, instead of coconut oil you can use three tablespoons of melted ghee per day. You can consume the coconut oil or ghee plain or mixed with half a cup of warm goat's or sheep's milk.

Coconut oil is best taken 20 minutes before each meal, as it will reduce appetite and help you feel full more quickly so that you will be satisfied with smaller portions. If you are under 180 pounds, take one tablespoon. If you are over 180 pounds, take two tablespoons. Alternatively, you can cook your foods with coconut oil or use it to make homemade salad dressings.

Purchase a high-quality, pure, organic, extra virgin, 100-percent coconut oil from the health food store or online. High-quality virgin coconut oil should be snow white in color when it is solid and water clear when it is liquid. If you see any shade of yellow or gray, the oil is of an inferior quality. Low-quality, non-virgin coconut oil is refined, bleached and deodorized, and contains contaminates.

Coconut oil is more effective for a weight-loss plan than olive oil.[321] Unlike long-chain fatty acids (LCFAs), the medium-chain fatty acids (MCFAs) in coconut oil are not deposited in fat depots in the body.[322]

Coconut oil is much purer than olive oil. Research has found that olive oil is adulterated with other oils. Adulterated olive oil has become the biggest source of agricultural fraud problems in the European Union. Less than 10 percent of the world's olive oil production meets the criteria for labeling as "extra virgin." Many olive oil brands labeled "extra virgin" are diluted with cheaper oils or vegetable oils that, when heated, cause disease. It's best to avoid olive oil unless you are 100 percent sure of its purity and quality.

ORGANIC TEA

Drinking tea daily helps prevent various diseases.[323] [324] Drinking between one and six cups of tea per day provides the most health benefits.[325] Tea contains catechins, a type of antioxidant that provides protection against disease. Green and black teas are especially high in catechins.

The consumption of green tea may be effective in preventing cancer.[326] It helps prevent cancer of the breast, esophagus, stomach, pancreas, and colon.[327] It is also effective in preventing and fighting heart disease, liver disease, Parkinson's disease, diabetes, and inflammatory bowel disease (IBD).[328]

Matcha green tea has higher concentrations of catechins than other types of green tea. Buddhist monks have drunk matcha green tea for centuries because it helps foster focused attention and alertness for meditation.

There's a difference between the caffeine found in coffee and the caffeine found in matcha green tea. Matcha green tea contains tannin, which slows the absorption of caffeine into the bloodstream. This means that the caffeine from matcha green tea is released gradually over the course of six to eight hours, unlike the short burst from coffee. Matcha green tea also contains two special amino acids called theophylline and L-theanine. L-theanine helps create a state of mental alertness while at the same time keeping you relaxed.[329]

Not only does matcha green tea boost mental alertness, it helps prevent cancer and heart disease,[330] making it the healthiest beverage to consume daily. An ancient Chinese proverb says that it is "better to be deprived of food for three days than tea for one."

Pu-erh (Yunnan Tuocha) tea is very high in antioxidants.[331] [332] In China, Pu-erh tea is widely believed to counteract the unpleasant effects of heavy alcohol consumption. It is traditionally used to strengthen the spleen and stomach as well as remove toxins from the body, improve eyesight, and promote blood circulation.

Researchers found that white tea had more catechins than many other types of tea.[333] Green and black teas undergo fermentation after harvest while white tea is unfermented.

Therefore, white tea has the highest concentration of antioxidants.

Drinking fennel tea after meals is very beneficial, as it is one of the most effective natural aids for digestion. It promotes the functioning of the kidneys, liver, and spleen.

Nettle tea is rich in nutrients, natural antihistamines, and anti-inflammatory substances. It is a powerful blood purifier. Herbalists use nettle to treat a wide variety of illnesses.

ORGANIC COFFEE

The caffeine in coffee is a stimulant that increases alertness, energy, and concentration, and is beneficial for treating fatigue.[334][335]

There is little evidence of health risks and much scientific evidence supporting the health benefits of moderate coffee consumption (three to four cups per day).[336]

Several studies have found that moderate coffee consumption may help prevent diseases such as certain types of cancer, type 2 diabetes, Parkinson's disease, Alzheimer's disease, and liver disease.[337] Research suggests that there is an ingredient in coffee that protects against liver cirrhosis.[338] Those drinking four cups of coffee per day had an 84 percent lower risk of cirrhosis,[339] a 67 percent lower risk of developing diabetes,[340] a 42 percent lower risk of liver cancer,[341] and a 57 percent reduced risk of (non-hormone-responsive) breast cancer.[342] A meta-analysis found that regular coffee drinkers had a reduced risk of bladder, breast, buccal, pharyngeal, colorectal, endometrial, esophageal, hepatocellular, leukemic, pancreatic, and prostate cancers.[343] A meta-analysis found that coffee intake is associated with a reduced risk of endometrial cancer.[344] Those who consumed four cups of coffee per day had a 25 percent lower risk of endometrial cancer than did those who consumed less than one cup per day. However, the addition of sugar and cream to coffee could counteract any potential benefits.[345]

Drinking coffee can raise blood pressure briefly, right after consumption.[346] However, a 15-year study of more than 41,000 people found that the risk of death from cardiovascular disease was 24 percent lower among those consuming one to three cups of coffee daily.[347]

A study based on a major European investigation into the effects of diet and lifestyle on health found that people who drank four or more cups of coffee a day were at no higher risk for chronic disease than were those who drank less than a cup of coffee a day.[348]

Many holistic health experts and naturopathic physicians have no major concerns with moderate coffee consumption but are against heavy coffee consumption. Naturopaths warn that heavy coffee consumption can lead to adrenal gland exhaustion, digestive disorders, nutrient deficiency, acidic body pH, and dehydration. Naturopaths also warn about the chemicals found in coffee. Coffee is also one of the most heavily chemically sprayed crops. There are more carcinogens in a single cup of coffee than carcinogenic pesticide residues in the average American diet in a year.[349] These chemicals burden the liver so that it is less able to detoxify toxins. Therefore, purchase only organic coffee.

For those who would like to limit their coffee intake, coffee substitutes such as Cafix, Dandy Blend, or maca root are available. Both Cafix and Dandy Blend have a similar—if not identical—taste to coffee. There are also other coffee substitutes you can try, such as Inka, Teeccino, Pero, Ayurvedic Roast, and Kaffree Roma, which are made with ingredients such as rye, barley, and chicory. Most coffee substitutes taste very similar to coffee.

Cafix is made in Poland and has a taste that is very close to coffee. It is made from barley, chicory, figs, and red beet extract. You can also mix organic coffee with Cafix in a 50 percent ratio to reduce your intake of caffeine.

Dandy Blend is made from dandelion roots, chicory, beets, barley, and rye. Dandy Blend is an instant beverage with a lot of essential minerals. Dandelion root has many beneficial health effects, such as improving digestion and detoxifying the liver.

Maca root powder doesn't taste like coffee but has the same energy-boosting effects. Maca root powder can be added to a fruit smoothie or protein shake. Maca is also available in the form of an instant beverage known as maca coffee, which has a coffee-like flavor.

SUPER SPICES

Super spices and herbs are high in antioxidants and rich in phytonutrients, such as carotenoids, flavonoids, and other phenolics, which possess health-promoting properties. "Some herbs should be considered as regular vegetables," says Shiow Y. Wang, PhD., a researcher and biochemist. "People should use more herbs for flavoring instead of salt and artificial chemicals." Using more herbs and spices is a good way to start eating healthier because, with the added flavor, you can reduce the salt and sugar in your recipes.

The capsaicin in peppers has a thermogenic effect, which boosts metabolism. Researchers suggest that adding three chili peppers to your diet will increase calorie burning after a meal and stimulate fat burning.[350] You can use red pepper in its various forms (cayenne, crushed red pepper, paprika) to spice up hummus, cottage cheese, guacamole, meat, fish, whole grain dishes, sauces, dips, and vinaigrettes.

Throughout the Orient, turmeric is traditionally used for both prevention of and therapy for diseases. Turmeric, derived from the plant Curcuma longa, is a gold-colored spice commonly used in India. Curcumin, a substance in turmeric, has been shown to exhibit antioxidant, anti-inflammatory, antiviral, antibacterial, antifungal, and anticancer activities and has the potential to treat various cancers, diabetes, allergies, arthritis, Alzheimer's disease, and other chronic illnesses.[351]

Oregano is very high in antioxidants.[352] Studies have shown that the herb's antioxidant power has 42 times more antioxidant activity than apples, 30 times more than potatoes, 12 times more than oranges, and four times more than blueberries.[353] One teaspoon has as much antioxidant power as three cups of chopped broccoli. It is effective for cancer prevention and has been shown to kill cancer cells.[354]

Oregano can be added seamlessly into familiar, everyday foods such as homemade pasta or pizza sauces, sandwiches, meats, fish, and whole grain dishes.

Dr. Richard A. Anderson of the U.S. Agriculture Department's Beltsville Human Nutrition Research Center has shown that taking the equivalent of one-quarter to one-half a teaspoon of cinnamon twice a day lowered glucose, total cholesterol, LDL-C, and triglyceride levels by up to 30 percent. Cinnamon is highly effective at helping stabilize blood sugar levels, making it ideal for those with diabetes.[355] One teaspoon of ground cinnamon has the equivalent level of antioxidants as a half cup of blueberries and one cup of pomegranate juice. You can put one teaspoon into your coffee grinds before brewing or stir into your honey to sweeten any beverage. You can also add cinnamon to yogurt, oatmeal, or smoothies.

Cumin, like cinnamon, helps keep blood sugar levels stable, which means cumin is great for diabetics or pre-diabetics. Cumin was found to be more effective than glibenclamide, an antidiabetic drug, in the treatment of diabetes mellitus.[356]

Cloves have been measured as having the highest antioxidant level of all spices and herbs.[357] Cloves help with digestive problems like gas, indigestion, nausea, and vomiting, and eliminate harmful parasites, bacteria, and fungi in the digestive system.

Parsley is used by diabetics in Turkey to reduce blood glucose. It has been shown to lower levels of blood glucose and has a hepato-protective effect.[358] Parsley contains apigenin, an antioxidant compound that possesses anti-inflammatory, antioxidant, and anticancer properties. Apigenin has also been found to protect against cancer, improve cardiovascular health, and stimulate the immune system.[359]

SEA SALT

Consumption of refined table salt has been linked to many diseases, including high blood pressure, cardiovascular disease, kidney disease, stroke, osteoporosis, and stomach cancer.[360 361 362 363 364 365] High sodium intake leads to a greater likelihood of being overweight and obese.[366 367 368]

Eliminate from your diet unhealthy sources of sodium, such as fast foods, chips, and commercially prepared baked goods and sweets. Replace table salt with unrefined sea salt, a healthy source of sodium. Completely eliminating sodium from your diet is not recommended and increases the prevalence of type 2 diabetes[369 370] and atherosclerosis.[371]

The best and purest commercially available salt is Himalayan salt and unrefined Celtic sea salt harvested from the Atlantic seawater off the coast of Brittany, France. Celtic sea salt contains all of the 84 beneficial minerals, with no chemicals, preservatives, or other additives.

Buy Celtic sea salt or Himalayan salt whenever you can; otherwise, the next best choice is unrefined sea salt. There are many brands of sea salt, so make sure you purchase the best quality. Real sea salt should not be pure white and powdery like refined table salt. Real sea salt has color and texture to it.

HOT IONIZED WATER

Drinking hot or warm water first thing in the morning and before meals is very beneficial. It reduces metabolic waste and improves digestion and elimination. "The consumption of warm water increases the tightening of the intestines, which optimizes elimination," explains Stella Metsovas, clinical nutritionist and health expert. Metsovas recommends drinking only hot water—and not cold water—before meals, as cold water reduces digestive power.

You can conduct a deep digestive and lymphatic system cleanse for several months by daily drinking "hot ionized water" that has been boiled for 20 minutes. Keep it in a Thermos and take a few sips every half an hour or more often. To have a powerful cleansing effect, the water must be boiled for at least 20 minutes and consumed as hot as you would drink tea. This hot water cleanse will flush toxins from your body.

When you boil water for 20 minutes, it becomes charged and saturated with negative oxygen ions. When you take frequent sips of this water throughout the day, it begins to thoroughly cleanse body tissues and help rid them of certain positively charged ions (associated with harmful acids and toxins).

Most toxins and waste materials carry a positive charge and, thus, tend to attach themselves to the body, which is negatively charged overall. As the negative oxygen ions enter the body with the ingested water, they are attracted to the positively charged toxic material. This neutralizes wastes and toxins, turning them into fluid matter that the body can easily remove. "The sipping of hot ionized water has a profound cleansing effect on all the tissues of the body," explains Andreas Moritz, a medical intuitive and practitioner of Ayurveda, iridology, and vibrational medicine.[372]

Drinking "hot ionized water" every day for several weeks or several months will help you lose weight. "If you have excessive body weight, this cleansing method can help you shed many pounds of body waste in a short period of time, without the side effects that normally accompany sudden weight loss," says Moritz.

LEMON WATER

Drinking a glass of warm water and the juice of half a freshly squeezed lemon every day will help you lose body fat, prevent weight gain, and reduce food cravings.[373]

Besides weight loss, lemon water provides numerous health benefits. Lemon water improves digestion, cleanses your body, boosts immunity, and improves energy levels. Lemons are rich in vitamins, minerals, dietary fibers, essential oils, and carotenoids.[374]

PURE WATER

Drinking plenty of pure water is essential for successful weight loss. The human body is approximately 57 to 75 percent water, depending on age.[375] Ultrapure water should be used for drinking, cooking, tea/coffee water, and bathing/showering.

Drinking tap water should be avoided at all costs. Tap water contains a multitude of poisonous chemicals and contaminants that are linked to millions of instances of illness. A report by the Ralph Nader Study Group stated, "U.S. drinking water contains more than two thousand toxic chemicals that can cause cancer."[376] The U.S. Council on Environmental Quality said, "Cancer risk among people drinking chlorinated water is as much as 93 percent higher than among those whose water does not contain chlorine." Scientific evidence shows a link between consumption of toxins in drinking water and elevated cancer risk.[377]

According to an analysis of federal data from *The New York Times*, more than 20 percent of the water treatment systems in the United States have violated key provisions of the Safe Drinking Water Act over the last five years. Tap water has contained illegal concentrations of chemicals like arsenic or radioactive substances like uranium, as well as dangerous bacteria often found in sewage. Many of the most dangerous illegal concentrations of contaminants regulated by the Safe Drinking Water Act have been tied to diseases like cancer that can take years to develop. In some U.S. cities, drinking water tests have detected illegal concentrations of arsenic, radioactive elements, and the dry cleaning solvent tetrachloroethylene, all of which have been linked to cancer. Millions of Americans may become ill every year due to the parasites, viruses, and bacteria in drinking water.[378]

Bottled water is not much better than tap water. An independent test by the Environmental Working Group found arsenic, disinfection byproducts (DPBs), and 36 other harmful pollutants in bottled water. Plastic bottles can contain the chemical Bisphenol A (BPA), which leaches into the water and has been found to be harmful to one's health.[379]

With all the different types of water filtration systems out there, it's easy to get confused about which filter provides the purest water and is best for your health.

The purest water is triple-distilled water. Distilled water has been put through the process of distillation once, while triple-distilled water has been put through the process of distillation three times.

Peter A. Lodewick, MD, author of *A Diabetic Doctor Looks at Diabetes*, says, "Distillation is the single most effective method of water purification." Distillation, when combined with carbon filtration, will kill and remove 99.9 percent of bacteria, viruses, and cysts, as well as heavy metals and volatile organic compounds. Reverse osmosis is the next best water filtration system. Reverse osmosis, when combined with carbon filtration, provides drinking water that is 98 to 99 percent free of chemicals.

Ionic adsorption micron filters are an affordable way to get ultrapure water available through a family water pitcher, filtration travel bottle, or water straw. Ionic adsorption micro filtration removes up to 99.99 percent of contaminants and pollutants such as bacteria, viruses, chemicals, heavy metals, and chlorine. The ionic adsorption micron filter (BPA- and lead-free) water bottle is great for travelers, campers, hikers, and those constantly on the move. It can be used with any type of water source: tap or rainwater, rivers, streams, and even lakes (excluding salt water).

Ultrapure water can be ozonated to make it even purer and to turn it into a healing substance.[380] Ozone destroys viruses, bacteria, parasites, and fungi.

In the human body, there are two types of water: bound water and structured water. Bound water becomes physically bound to other molecule structures and is unable to freely move through the cell wall. It lingers around the cell, causing bloating and water retention.

Scientists in Korea and Japan have studied the health benefits of altered water and have found it to be superior to regular filtered water. However, scientists in Western countries have not thoroughly studied altered water.

Structured water—also known as hexagonal water or microclustered water—is an altered water that has smaller clusters than regular water, allowing for much better absorption and hydration than regular filtered water. Among those with diabetes, structured water has been shown to lower blood sugar levels in just four weeks.[381] It also strengthens the immune system, increasing lymphocyte production.[382]

Aging is caused by a loss of structured water from organs, tissues, and cells, and an overall decrease in total body water.[383] Therefore, drinking structured water could delay the aging process.

Dr. Gerald Pollack has been doing research on water in his laboratory at the University of Washington for years. He has found that structured water is the best type of water you can drink to promote health.

Structured water is essential for health because it is water in an optimal, balanced state. Structured water strengthens the immune system, rehydrates the body faster and more effectively than regular water, and increases energy levels. It also tastes better than regular water.

The "healing water" from the Ganges and Lourdes has been studied and found to have the signature of the structured water found in cells.

The absolute best water to drink is water that has been filtered and then poured into a water structuring bottle or structuring cup. Whether you use reverse osmosis, distillation, ozonation, or an ionic adsorption micron filter, after filtration the water is frequently de-structured.

Electrolyzed reduced water or alkaline-reduced water (ARW) is another type of altered water that is especially useful for healing illness. Research has shown that it has anticancer, antidiabetic, and anti-aging effects. It has been shown to reduce glucose, triglyceride, and cholesterol levels.[384] [385] [386] It has also been shown to delay tumor growth and to lengthen lifespans.[387]

Drinking lots of water is commonly considered part of a weight-loss regimen. Water induces thermogenesis, and drinking 1,500 milliliters of water per day has been shown to decrease body weight, BMI, and body composition. Research suggests that drinking 500 milliliters of water half an hour before each meal boosts metabolism and decreases the amount of food eaten.[388 389 390]

Although there is plenty of research showing the health benefits of drinking water, many people don't like the taste of it or find it boring to drink.

Infused water—also called detox water—is filtered water flavored with fruits and herbs that satisfy many people's taste buds and offer additional weight-loss benefits as compared to plain water. You can use blueberries, raspberries, blackberries, strawberries, watermelon pieces, tangerine slices, orange slices, grapefruit slices, lemon slices, lime slices, mango pieces, cucumber slices, fresh mint, fresh basil, cinnamon sticks, and fresh ginger slices. You can also add organic coconut water to contribute even more flavor.

Experiment with various infused water recipes and see how many fruit slices or herbs you need to be satisfied with the taste of the water. Some of the most common infused water recipes are:

- Lemon cucumber water
- Lemon, watermelon, and mint water
- Apple cinnamon water
- Mango ginger water
- Orange strawberry water
- Blueberry orange water
- Green apple, cucumber, and mint water

You can also drink apple cider vinegar diluted in water for a tangy flavor. Dilute one to two tablespoons in a big glass of water and sip it along with your meals one or two times a day.

CHAPTER SUMMARY

- Eat a balanced, healthy diet based on the Weston Price diet or the Mediterranean diet. Eat foods low on the GI and GL, and foods with a high satiety index. Divide your plate in the following way at each meal: one-half vegetables, one-quarter whole grains or starches, and one-quarter protein.

- Eat from every essential food group and include a variety of healthy foods in your diet, including organic fruits and vegetables; organic whole grains and pulses, prepared properly; unroasted organic nuts and seeds; fresh shellfish; wild-caught fish; fish eggs; insects; 100-percent grass-fed meat, wild game, and organ meats; free-range, organic eggs; healthy fats; lacto-fermented foods and beverages; unpasteurized, unhomogenized, grass-fed, raw, organic dairy; unrefined Celtic or Himalayan sea salt; apple cider or rice vinegar; and super spices.

- Enjoy desserts made with low GI flours such as coconut flour, quinoa flour, oat flour, spelt flour, kamut flour, rye flour, barley flour, or buckwheat flour, and use natural sweeteners such as pure stevia, coconut palm sugar, sugarcane juice, maple syrup, Manuka honey, and blackstrap molasses. By using low GI sweeteners and low GI flours you can enjoy dessert whenever you feel like it and never restrict yourself, because the key to long-term weight loss is not restricting yourself.

- The absolute best water to drink is water that has been filtered with reverse osmosis, distillation, ozonation, or an ionic adsorption micron filter, and, after filtration, altered into structured water or electrolyzed reduced water. Make fruit-infused water so that the beverage is palatable to your taste buds.

- Have only homemade bone broth soup for dinner or nothing at all. Consuming bone broth soup for "souper" will help you sleep better. Make homemade bone broth by boiling the bones of grass-fed cattle, bison, free-range poultry, or wild-caught fish.

CHAPTER 3

LIFESTYLE

It's not new information that if you want to get healthier and lose weight permanently, you need to make exercise a regular part of your life. To get rid of excess weight, you must exercise and follow a proper diet. Numerous studies show that exercise alone or diet alone will not lead to satisfactory weight loss.[1]

Successful weight loss through exercise is dependent on the circadian rhythm, as is every other factor in a healthy lifestyle. Researchers have found that the timing of exercise is an important factor for those who lose weight in response to exercise. Exercising at the wrong time—at night—can disrupt the circadian rhythm. This explains why some people do not lose weight when they exercise at night.[2]

BENEFITS OF EXERCISE

Exercise is extremely important for the maintenance of good health and the prevention of disease. "Those who think they have not time for bodily exercise will sooner or later have to find time for illness," said English statesman Edward Stanley. Increased frequency of exercise was associated with reduced risk of death.[3] Those who exercise more frequently live longer.[4] Improving fitness can reduce the risk of death by 44 percent.[5]

American cartoonist Randy Glasbergen said, "What fits your busy schedule better, exercising one hour a day or being dead twenty-four hours a day?" Regular exercise decreases the risk of cardiovascular disease, type 2 diabetes, osteoporosis, and colon and breast cancer. Exercise has been shown to improve insulin sensitivity, reduce blood pressure, reduce inflammation, and decrease blood coagulation.[6]

Regular exercise slows aging.[7] "We do not stop exercising because we grow old—we grow old because we stop exercising," said Dr. Kenneth H. Cooper, MD. Exercise is a natural anti-aging therapy. A lack of exercise actually speeds up the aging process.[8] Chronic stress is known to accelerate aging. However, exercise can buffer the impact of stress on aging.[9]

Aerobic exercise is known to strengthen and enlarge the heart muscle, which improves the efficiency with which it pumps, resulting in better circulation. Better circulation results in better health. American athlete Jack LaLanne said, "Yes, exercise is the catalyst. That's what makes everything happen: your digestion, your elimination, your sex life, your skin, hair, everything about you depends on circulation."

Exercise promotes positive change in all aspects of health, whether physically, emotionally, or mentally. "Movement is a medicine for creating change in a person's physical, emotional, and mental states," said Carol Welch, founder of BioSomatics Education, a method that supports the body's capacity to be posturally functional by overcoming neuromuscular conditions.

AMOUNT OF EXERCISE

The American College of Sports Medicine recommends 60 to 90 minutes of moderate activity per day. At a minimum, three hours per week of regular aerobic (cardio) exercise is the suggested amount required to lose weight and keep it off. The greatest reduction in weight is likely to happen if you exercise between three hours and seven hours per week.[10]

Fast walking, jogging, swimming, cycling, rebounding (using a mini-trampoline), jumping rope, climbing stairs, playing tennis, dancing, and rowing are common forms of cardio exercises. Those who expend a higher percentage of calories through exercise do so through high-intensity activities such as jogging, cycling, and weight-lifting.[11]

Balancing the amount of exercise you perform is very important. Excessive endurance exercise is not better than no exercise at all. Numerous studies have shown that very strenuous endurance exercise damages the heart.[12]

The Copenhagen City Heart Study conducted a study on healthy joggers between 20 and 86 years of age who were followed for 12 years to compare the long-term all-cause mortality rates among light, moderate, and strenuous joggers. They found that people who jog lightly and moderately for one to two hours per week have lower mortality than sedentary people who don't jog at all, whereas those who jog more than four hours per week, at a very fast pace, have a mortality rate not much different from that of the sedentary group. The researchers found that the optimal frequency of jogging is two to three times per week at a slow or average pace for a length of up to two and a half hours per week.[13]

Studies have found that long-term training for and competition in extreme endurance events such as marathons, Ironman distance triathlons, and very long distance bicycle races cause heart damage in healthy individuals.[14]

RAPID FAT LOSS EXERCISE

Most exercise programs aimed at fat loss focus on exercises such as walking and jogging at a moderate intensity. However, moderate-intensity exercise does not lead to satisfactory weight loss for the majority of people.[15 16]

Interval-type exercise is more beneficial for weight loss than many hours of strenuous endurance-type exercise. Weight loss achieved during very strenuous exercise tends to get reversed because the body tries to quickly replenish its fat stores, as it perceives marathon-type exercise as a threat to survival.[17]

Research has shown that high-intensity intermittent exercise (HIIE), also called sprint interval training (SIT), or high-intensity interval training (HIT), is the most effective type of exercise for reducing body fat rapidly, as well as reducing blood pressure, triglycerides, and fasting glucose.[18 19]

High-intensity exercise promotes fat breakdown more than moderate-intensity exercise does because of the release of certain hormones (PGC-1 and BAIBA), which increase calorie burning.[20]

The American College of Sports Medicine reports that you can raise your metabolism for up to 24 hours post-exercise by doing high-intensity intermittent exercise. A study found that a single session of high-intensity intermittent exercise increases calorie burning by over 200 calories post-workout.[21]

The additional benefit of high-intensity intermittent exercise is that it achieves health and weight-loss results in a shorter amount of time than do other forms of cardio exercise programs.

High-intensity intermittent exercise typically involves sprinting or pedaling as fast as possible, followed immediately by low-intensity exercise or resting six seconds to four minutes.

Cycling on a stationary bicycle is one way to do high-intensity exercise for rapid fat loss. Pedal at maximum speed on a stationary bicycle for a set amount of time.

The Wingate test is a good exercise program to follow if you have the right motivation and a high fitness level. The Wingate test consists of 30 seconds of hardcore pedaling with hard resistance. It's typically performed four to six times, separated by four minutes of rest. This protocol amounts to around four minutes of exercise per session, with each session typically performed three times a week for two to six weeks.[22]

An easier interval workout involves pedaling as fast as possible on a stationary bike for 30 seconds with five sprints in total, each sprint separated by four minutes of recovery and slow pedaling.

A less demanding exercise program that may be suitable for most people consists of eight seconds of high-intensity cycling followed by 12 seconds of low-intensity cycling for a period of 20 minutes.[23]

Another easy eight-minute interval workout involves four one-minute sets of jumping jacks done as fast as you comfortably can, with one minute of rest between each set.

You can design your own interval workout based on the types of exercises you like to do. All you have to do is inject brief periods of intense effort into your workouts, whether they are running, swimming, bicycling, elliptical sessions, etc.

If you do not have a good fitness level, start by walking for 30 minutes. Then try adding a burst of jogging for 30 seconds every five minutes. As you increase your fitness level, you can increase the interval length to a minute and decrease the walking to four minutes.

Bouts of high-intensity activity raise your metabolism rapidly, and your body continues to burn calories at an accelerated rate even after your workout is over. For the biggest metabolism boost, make sure that the interval portion leaves you breathing hard.

The best time for high-intensity intermittent exercise is in the morning, on an empty stomach, before breakfast (fasted cardio).[24] A study found that when people fasted during morning cardio they burned 20 percent more fat than when they had a meal before exercise.[25]

High-intensity intermittent fasted cardio in the morning is effective in rapidly burning fat. That's because as you fast overnight your body conserves its carb stores, so in the morning your body is geared toward mobilizing fat for fuel. Fasted cardio seems to work especially well for people who want to eliminate resistant or stubborn fat areas on their bodies.[26]

A benefit of fasted cardio in the morning is that you will burn calories for the rest of the day, even when you're not doing anything. Even though slow or moderate cardio burns more total calories and fat during the actual workout, the high-intensity intermittent cardio program leads to greater total fat loss because it burns more calories and fat the rest of the day, which adds up to more calories and fat than you can burn during a single workout session.

BUILD MUSCLE MASS

Your body burns calories at rest. The number of calories your body burns at rest is called your resting metabolic rate (RMR). Your RMR is the number of calories you require to maintain your body's weight if you did not move all day.

A pound of muscle burns more calories per day than a pound of fat does. The more muscle you build, the more calories your body will burn all day long. For each pound of muscle gained, you'll burn about six to ten calories per day.[27] Cedric Bryant, PhD, the chief science officer for the American Council on Exercise (ACE), states that muscle burns roughly 7 to 10 calories per pound per day, compared to two to three calories per pound per day for fat.

You need to build muscle mass if you are reducing your calorie intake so that you lose body fat without losing muscle. The best thing about losing weight through weight training is that you will lose only fat mass. Cardio tends to make you lose muscle mass along with fat.

The best tools for weight training are adjustable dumbbells, as you can do almost any type of exercise with them. You can use them to target every major muscle in the body. Full body high-intensity intermittent training (HIIT) with weights is the best fat burning exercise. To design your exercise program, choose some compound exercises that will target all the primary muscles of your body. Compound exercises utilize multiple joints with free weights.

- Squats
- Deadlifts
- Arnold press
- Dumbbell rows with both hands
- Clean and press
- Push up row
- Lunges

If you want to select only six basic movements to target every muscle, you can choose from among the following:

- Horizontal push and pull
- Vertical push and pull
- Hip dominant
- Quad dominant

For all the mentioned movements, it's best to hire a personal trainer to help you do them correctly. You can divide these upper body and lower body movements so that you do them two times each per week. For example, on Monday do lower body, on Tuesday do upper body, on Thursday do lower body, and on Friday or Saturday do upper body.[28]

It's essential to set up your weight training routine in a way that ensures a balance around the joints (shoulders, knees, elbows) and balance between the different movement patterns (horizontal push/pull, vertical push/pull) to prevent injury and build a balanced-looking body.[29]

Learning to properly weight train to build a balanced-looking, attractive body and to prevent injury is a topic that needs a book of its own. You can learn a lot from a good personal trainer, by watching videos, and by reading and participating in bodybuilding forums such as Body Building (www.bodybuilding.com).

KEEP WEIGHT OFF

Research shows that there's one thing regular, moderate exercise is really good at, and that's preventing weight regain. Once you have reached your ideal weight through high-intensity exercise, you need to perform moderate intensity exercise and follow certain lifestyle habits to keep the weight off.

The National Weight Control Registry (NWCR) is a research study that includes adults who have lost at least 13.6 kg (30 pounds) of weight and kept it off for at least one year. On average, those in the study have lost an average of 66 pounds and kept it off for 5.5 years. There are currently more than 10,000 people enrolled in the study, making it the largest study of successful weight loss maintenance ever conducted. It's not surprising that 98 percent of people have reduced their food intake, 94 percent have increased their exercise, and 90 percent exercise for about one hour per day. After losing weight, almost all of the participants ate breakfast and weighed themselves about once per week. They watch less television than the average American, which leaves time to engage in moderate intensity exercise.[30] Women in the study consume an average of 1,306 calories per day; men consume 1,685 calories per day.[31]

MAKE EXERCISING EASY

The biggest problem that many people have is a lack of motivation, energy, time, or consistent long-term dedication to exercise. You need to create an environment that leaves little room for excuses.

In his book *The Magic of Thinking Big*, David Schwartz coined the word "excusitis" (from the root word "excuse"), which is defined as "the disease of the failures." It's a behavior of a person who finds all sorts of excuses to justify his or her poor results or lack of action. Some common excuses for not exercising include: "I don't have the time," "I don't have the energy," "Exercising is boring," "I'm too old," and "I'm in pain."

The only way to cure "excusitis" is to take action. Therefore, instead of making excuses take action and take steps toward your goal of weight loss. Successful weight loss is a journey that requires persistence, endurance, and no room for excuses. For the majority of people, the hardest part is starting. As humans, we naturally look for the path of least resistance.

Lying to yourself seems to work. If you tell yourself that you will go running for only five minutes, once you get going you may feel like running for a little longer.

Arrange your schedule and workout gear in such a way that you get into the habit of working out regularly. Eliminate barriers that prevent you from exercising. For example, always have your gym bag ready by the front door so that as soon as you leave your home, all you have to do is grab it and go. Maybe you can move exercise equipment into your home or work office. Maybe you can talk on the phone while you exercise. To the extent that you can, replace driving with walking or biking.

Do whatever it takes to make exercise time-efficient and easy. Combining work and exercise avoids the need to find the time to exercise. If you don't have the time, you will never find the time. You need to make time by adding exercise into your daily life.

Exercise equipment is available that allows you to exercise comfortably while working and using your laptop. There is the DeskCycle, which is an under-desk pedal that allows you to pedal while sitting at your desk.

If you have a hectic life and forget to exercise then set up exercise and weight equipment in your home. You can attach a portable pull-up bar to the door outside your bedroom and every time you pass by you can do some pull-ups. In this way, you don't have to remember to do pull-ups, because you see the pull-up bar every time you walk into your bedroom.

Put your exercise routine into your schedule. If you need reminding, set up an alert on your calendar on your smartphone so that it reminds you automatically.

You can use an exercise diary app to keep track of the exercise you complete each week. By visually keeping track of the exercise you complete each week, you may be more motivated to reach your exercise goals each week.

Subscribe to a fitness magazine that you receive every month in the mail or on your tablet. The best magazines include the most recent scientific research on the topics of fitness, health, and bodybuilding. The best ones are *FitnessRX for Women* (www.fitnessrxwomen.com) and *FitnessRX for Men* (www.fitnessrxformen.com).

Even if you don't read the articles in your favorite fitness magazine, simply looking at the pictures of the fit, vibrant, healthy-looking, muscular men or women can motivate you to reach your fitness goals.

If you have a monthly subscription to a physical magazine, cut out a picture of your dream body and post it in your work area to serve as a visual reminder of your goal—one that you'll see every single day. For many people, visual reminders help them achieve their dream bodies.

One warning about magazines: Don't read the advertisements in any fitness magazine. Too many people have wasted their money on weight-loss or fat-burning pills that don't work, have no scientific validation or are even harmful to one's health.

If you don't have the energy or the desire to exercise, try to make exercise an enjoyable experience, a way to blow off steam, reduce stress levels, socialize, or listen to your favorite music.

Find an exercise buddy or hire a personal trainer and you'll be motivated to show up for a duration of exercise. A study conducted at the University of Pennsylvania School of Medicine proved that exercising with a partner improves weight-loss results.

There are websites that can help you find an exercise buddy, such as Exercise Friends (http://exercisefriends.com) or Workout Buddies Meetups (http://workout-buddies.meetup.com). You can also post an ad in a free online classifieds listing website stating that you are looking for a workout partner.

Researchers have found that different exercise environments have different effects on a person's mood and energy levels. They found that music and social contact enhanced mood and enjoyment during exercise.[32]

They found that people enjoy exercising outdoors more than they do indoors, and were less tense and stressed when exercising outdoors as compared to those who exercised indoors.

People had higher energy levels, were less tired, and enjoyed themselves when listening to music with a fast (as opposed to slow) tempo while exercising.

Exercise produces positive psychological and mood benefits, and these benefits are enhanced with music and social contact. When you exercise, your body releases chemicals called endorphins. These endorphins interact with the receptors in your brain that reduce your perception of pain. Endorphins act as analgesics, which mean they diminish the perception of pain.

If you set up your exercise environment in such a way that it makes you enjoy exercising, you can get a feeling known as "runner's high," which provides a positive and energizing outlook on life.

Regular exercise has been proven to reduce stress, boost self-esteem, improve sleep, increase energy levels, and reduce anxiety. Research has shown that exercise is an effective treatment for mild to moderate depression.[33]

Exercise should be fun and enjoyable, so select an activity you enjoy. Vary your exercises so that you don't get bored. There are so many different ways to move your body.

Rebounding, which consists of jumping on a mini trampoline, is one of the most effective types of exercise for improving health because of the effect it has on the lymph.[34] Research comparing rebounding exercise to treadmill jogging found no significant difference between the benefits of these two exercises.[35] However, the main benefit of rebounding is low trauma to the joints. Rebounding is a good alternative for those who have joint problems or have been told to avoid high-impact exercise.[36]

Swimming is a low-impact exercise, as it places no pressure on the joints. Regular swimming builds endurance, muscle strength, cardiovascular fitness, posture, and flexibility. However, be sure to swim in a salt-water pool, ozone-filtered pool, or natural pools of water like lakes and oceans. Swimming in chlorinated pools or sitting in a chlorinated hot tub may induce genotoxicity (DNA damage).[37] Carcinogenic byproducts have been detected in the blood of those swimming in chemically disinfected water.[38] You should also avoid steam rooms. Steam rooms are like toxic gas chambers. Use a dry sauna instead of a steam room.

It is extremely important to take a shower only in filtered water. Toxic chemicals evaporate out of the water and are inhaled.[39] Up to 100 times more toxic chemicals are taken in by showering than by drinking.[40] You can buy a shower filter online or at home stores.

Meditative movement (MM) is a type of exercise that has many proven health benefits. MM includes qigong, tai chi, and yoga. What classifies MM as different from traditional forms of exercise is the coordination of body, breath, and mind to achieve deep relaxation.[41] MM is classified as a mind-body intervention.

Qigong is a relaxing form of exercise with anti-aging benefits.[42] [43] Qigong means "working with the qi." Regular qigong practice is very beneficial for long-term health and longevity.[44] Qigong and tai chi are close relatives; however, qigong is designed for building health, while tai chi places more emphasis on the self-defense aspects of the training.

There is a wide range of health benefits in doing either qigong or tai chi. A comprehensive review of studies on qigong and tai chi found more than 100 different physiological and psychological health outcomes.[45]

Yoga is a combination of breathing exercises, physical postures, and meditation that has been practiced for thousands of years in India. Studies comparing the effects of yoga and exercise seem to indicate that yoga may be as effective as or even slightly more effective than exercise at improving a variety of health-related outcome measures.[46]

A study showed that practicing yoga improves cardiovascular function, reduces stress, improves sleep patterns, and enhances muscular strength and body flexibility.[47] An Indian study found that yoga treats and prevents heart disease.[48] Salivary cortisol (a measure of stress) decreased significantly after participation in a yoga class. Women also reported lower stress levels and anxiety after three months of practicing yoga.[49]

SPORTS DRINKS AND BARS

When you sweat during exercise, you lose water and electrolytes like sodium, potassium, magnesium, calcium, and chloride. It is very important to replenish electrolytes lost during exercise.

Electrolytes regulate our nerve and muscle function, our body's hydration, blood pH, blood pressure, and the rebuilding of damaged tissue. Low electrolyte levels can lead to either weak muscles, muscle cramps, twitching, irregular heartbeat, or fatigue. An electrolyte panel can be done as part of a routine physical to screen for any electrolyte imbalance.

Sports drinks designed to replenish electrolytes contain ingredients that promote weight gain and diabetes, such as high fructose corn syrup, sucrose syrup, and sugar. Both energy drinks and sports drinks can contain artificial additives, too much caffeine, and too much sugar.

If you are exercising regularly and working up a sweat, you can replenish electrolytes, hydrate, and energize with natural drinks like 100-percent pure coconut water. Coconut water replenishes body fluids better than do sports drinks.[50] Coconut water is low in calories, super hydrating, and very high in potassium (more potassium than four bananas). Coconut water has a sweet, nutty taste. If you are not a fan of coconut water, look for a sports drink that has a low GI and contains no artificial additives, and no high fructose corn syrup.

Many energy bars and meal replacement bars are high in calories and contain high fructose corn syrup, artificial sweeteners, and sugar. "Some [energy bars] are not much different than candy bars," says nutritionist Heidi Skolnik. "You really have to look at the label."

Look for "whole food" energy bars, protein bars, or meal replacement bars that are low GI and made from natural ingredients such as fruits, vegetables, nuts, seeds, and sprouted grains. They're typically sweetened naturally with real fruit or natural sweeteners such as stevia or honey. Many whole food energy bars are high in nutrients and fiber. Some high-quality energy or protein bars are raw and organic. Read the ingredient list to find an energy bar that's made with natural ingredients such as fruits, vegetables, nuts, seeds, and whole grains. Energy bars vary in taste, so try a few to find a brand that you like.

WEIGHING FREQUENTLY

Research shows that people who successfully lose weight and keep it off have higher levels of strenuous activity and weigh themselves more frequently.[51] The more often a person weighs himself or herself, the greater that person's 24-month weight-loss results and the less likely they are to regain weight in the long term if they continue to weigh themselves frequently.[52] Furthermore, a decline in the frequency of weighing is independently associated with weight regain.[53]

Weighing yourself, whether daily or weekly, provides an opportunity for positive reinforcement and motivation. Although some people believe weighing yourself regularly may negatively affect you, a study found that frequency of weighing was actually associated with a decline in depression, as well as increased self-control and motivation.[54]

In addition to weighing yourself, it's best to measure your body fat percentage to track your weight loss progress, especially if you are working on building muscle mass.

Weighing yourself will not show your progress accurately because one pound of fat weighs the same as one pound of muscle, although one pound of muscle occupies less space (volume) within the body than does one pound of fat.[55]

Body fat percentage is different for men than for women. Women have a higher body fat percentage relative to men on the same level. Women have more fat because of physical differences such as breasts. In addition, women need a higher amount of body fat for ovulation. A male athlete in superb shape will have about 10 percent body fat, while a woman at a comparable level of athleticism might be 18 to 20 percent body fat.[56]

Women should not have a body fat percentage below 17 percent if they are concerned about proper menstruation.[57] In the book *Taking Charge of Your Fertility*, Toni Weschler recommends a minimum body fat percentage of 18 while trying to conceive.

The ACE maintains one of the most commonly used body fat charts. Essential fat is the minimum amount of fat necessary for health.[58]

Body Fat Percent Norms for Men and Women		
Description	Women	Men
Essential Fat	10-13%	2-5%
Athletes	14-20%	6-13%
Fitness	21-24%	14-17%
Acceptable	25-31%	18-24%
Obesity	>32%	>25%

There are several ways to measure your body fat levels. Some methods are more accurate than others.[59]

Bioelectrical impedance analysis (BIA) is a commonly used method for estimating body composition, the measurement of body fat in relation to lean body mass. This non-invasive test involves the placement of two electrodes on the right hand and right foot. A low-level, imperceptible electrical current is sent through the body.

The Bod Pod is a space-age-looking machine that measures body fat composition, showing the percentage of your body that is fat and the percentage that is lean body mass. It works by measuring the volume of air you displace inside the pod, then runs it through a complicated mathematical equation to measure your fat, lean muscle mass, and resting metabolic rate.

A dual-energy X-ray absorptiometry (DEXA) scan is used primarily for measuring bone density. The scan consists of laying on a table and getting a full-body X-ray. You can get this done at a health facility.

Body fat scales and handheld devices are easy methods of measuring your body fat percentage, but are not as reliable and accurate as other methods; results vary depending on your hydration level.

Hydrostatic weighing—also referred to as underwater weighing or simply the dunk test—requires that you jump into a pool, sit on a stool, and get into a crunch position so that your body is completely underwater. You have to expel as much air as you possibly can, then hold perfectly still while the machine weighs you.

The InBody is a machine that measures your body fat percentage, where your fat is stored, and where you have water collecting in your body (edema), which can be a sign of injury or inflammation. It also measures your resting metabolic rate (RMR) and basal metabolic rate (BMR). It involves standing on a metal platform and holding onto two handles for about one minute. Most Lifetime Fitness gyms have this service available.

If you are going to start testing your body fat percentage, make sure to test yourself under the same conditions each and every time. For example every Monday morning, on a completely empty stomach—no food or drink.

RESTFUL SLEEP

Sleep is as essential as a good diet and exercise for weight loss and maintenance. The problem is that 35 to 40 percent of the adult U.S. population reports sleeping less than seven hours on weekday nights.[60] Many night-shift workers often struggle with weight loss because they have continued disruption of their circadian rhythms.

The old adage, "early to bed, early to rise, makes a man healthy, wealthy, and wise" stands up to the test of research. Lack of sleep (less than five hours) disrupts the circadian rhythm, causing weight gain, hypertension, and diabetes.[61 62 63 64] Even a few night shifts per week can throw off the circadian rhythm and increase the risk of obesity and type 2 diabetes.[65]

The International Agency for Research on Cancer concluded that shift work disrupts the circadian rhythm and is probably carcinogenic (cancer-causing) to humans.[66 67]

In the largest, most diverse study to date under controlled laboratory conditions, lack of sleep promoted weight gain. Chronically sleep-restricted adults with late bedtimes and who ate late at night are very susceptible to weight gain.[68]

In a study involving 21,469 healthy individuals aged 20 years or older, the individuals who slept less than five hours were more likely to experience weight gain than were those who slept seven hours per night.[69]

The largest and longest study to date on adult sleep habits and weight is the Nurses' Health Study, which followed 68,000 women for up to 16 years. The study found that those who slept five hours or less were more likely to become obese compared to those who slept seven hours per night.[70]

Scientists have discovered that overexposure to light, or light exposure during odd hours, leads to disruption of the circadian rhythm, causing weight gain and weight-related diseases, including type 2 diabetes and cardiovascular disease.

In the study, mice exposed to a prolonged day length of 16 and 24-hour light, compared with regular 12-hour light, gained weight even though their food intake or physical activity was unaffected.[71] The scientists concluded that prolonged exposure to light causes the body to store more calories rather than burn them.

Research demonstrates that any sort of light exposure at night (even the most minimal) increases body mass, disrupts core body temperature, and decreases fat metabolism.[72]

Remove any sort of light exposure that will disrupt your circadian rhythm, such as lights coming in from the bedroom window, an LED alarm clock by the bed, a television, a cell phone, or a battery-charging station with power light indicator buttons shining.

Adjust your sleep schedule according to the sunrise and sunset. Our ancestors did not have artificial light and went to sleep as soon as the sun set. It may take some time and effort to correct your sleep pattern, but it can be done with natural and effective remedies.

Research shows that the scent of lavender essential oil helps people fall asleep and sleep much better. Researchers at

Wesleyan University had people sniff lavender essential oil or distilled water (placebo) just before bedtime. The researchers monitored the subjects' sleep cycles with brain scans. When the study participants had sniffed lavender, they slept more soundly; they also felt more energetic the next morning.[73]

There are a few ways to use pure lavender essential oil. You can place a few drops on your wrists. You can sprinkle a few drops on a piece of tissue and tuck it under your pillow. You can also use an aromatherapy diffuser.

Take the time to design a bedroom environment that promotes deep sleep so that you wake up each morning feeling refreshed.

The National Sleep Foundation suggests dimming the lights about an hour before bed. Use room darkening shades and curtains to keep it dark at night and while you sleep. A cool room temperature between 60 and 67 degrees makes for the best sleep. Experiment with your room's exact temperature to find what makes you most comfortable.

The National Sleep Foundation conducted a two-year study to discover exactly how much sleep a person needs at each age:[74]

- Teenagers (14 to 17): Sleep range should be eight to ten hours
- Younger adults (18 to 25): Sleep range should be seven to nine hours
- Adults (26 to 64): Sleep range should be seven to nine hours
- Older adults (65+): Sleep range should be seven to eight hours

Many people don't consider sleep that important and prefer other activities that are considered more important and of greater value.[75] Work and commuting to and from work were the two activities most often exchanged for sleep.[76] If you really value your health, the way you look, and the way you feel, you will make sleep a top priority. You really need to schedule sleep like any other daily activity, so put it on your "to-do list" and cross it off every night.

Ideally, always go to sleep two hours before midnight. Really deep sleep lasts from 11 p.m. until midnight. If you skip this deep sleep period regularly, your body and mind become exhausted and your body will secrete stress hormones such as adrenaline and cortisol. Lack of sleep reduces growth hormone production, leading to weight gain. The less quality sleep you get, the more overweight you are likely to get.

If you have major problems with insomnia, consult a naturopath to help you deal with this issue and consider using nutritional support such as oral melatonin 1 mg around bedtime (short term only). Melatonin has been shown to be safe and effective in the treatment of insomnia and other circadian rhythm sleep disorders.[77]

Sleep with an eye mask every night. The release of the hormone melatonin is responsible for the feeling of sleepiness. It is released by the pineal gland, and production starts by exposure to darkness. Wearing an eye mask improves sleep quality and elevates melatonin levels.[78]

CHAPTER SUMMARY

- High-intensity intermittent exercise (HIIE), also called sprint interval training (SIT) or high-intensity interval training (HIT), is the most effective form of exercise for rapidly reducing body fat.

- The best time for high-intensity intermittent exercise is in the morning, on an empty stomach, before breakfast (fasted cardio) for no longer than 60 minutes.

- Full-body high-intensity intermittent training (HIIT) with weights is an excellent fat-burning exercise.

- The best tools for weight training are adjustable dumbbells, as you can do almost any type of exercise with them. You can use them to target every major muscle in the body.

- Once you have reached your ideal weight through high-intensity exercise, you must perform moderate intensity exercise regularly to keep the weight off.

- After exercise, replenish lost electrolytes with coconut water or a sports drink that has a low GI and that contains no artificial additives and no high fructose corn syrup. Choose "whole food" energy bars, protein bars, or meal replacement bars instead of high-sugar bars.

- Weigh yourself regularly, at least once per week, to stay motivated and keep track of your progress. In addition, measure your body fat levels regularly.

- Make time for exercise in your daily life and create an environment that leaves little room for excuses. Combine work and exercise. Use the DeskCycle, which is an under-desk pedal that allows you to pedal while sitting at your desk and working on your laptop.

- Do whatever it takes to make it time-efficient and easier for you to exercise. If you have a hectic life and forget to exercise, set up exercise and weight equipment in your home. Attach a portable pull-up bar to the door outside your bedroom and do some pull-ups every time you pass by it.

- Exercise should be fun and enjoyable, so select an activity you enjoy, blast some good music, and exercise with a friend to get that "runner's high."

- Vary your exercises so that you don't get bored. There are so many types of exercises with beneficial health effects, such as rebounding, swimming, meditative movement (MM), qigong and tai chi, and yoga.

- Make seven to nine hours of sleep a priority and use melatonin, an eye mask, and pure lavender essential oil to help you fall asleep. Go to sleep between 10 p.m. and 11 p.m., as really deep sleep lasts from 11 p.m. until midnight. Regularly skipping this prime time to sleep will cause your mind to become exhausted and your body to secrete stress hormones such as adrenaline and cortisol.

CHAPTER 4

SUPPLEMENTS

Nutrients and thermogenics are best derived from whole foods rather than from supplements. Nutrients from whole foods have been shown to be superior to synthetic vitamins or minerals.[1][2][3] Whenever possible, get your nutritional needs from whole foods. Sometimes, though, supplements are recommended. For example, they may be necessary when trying to eliminate stubborn body fat or when treating health conditions or nutritional deficiencies that hinder weight loss.

The next best thing to consuming whole foods is to take a whole food supplement. Whole food supplements are made from concentrated whole foods. A whole food supplement is absorbed and assimilated by the body better than synthetic supplements are.

Thermogenics increase metabolism and fat burning by increasing the heat in the body. They can help you quickly lose weight because they are designed to promote lipolysis in the body (the breaking down of body fat to be used as energy).

People who are used to frequent snacking and those who experience hunger between meals need an appetite suppressant to help them get to the next meal without snacking.

Appetite suppressants control feelings of hunger and promote the sense of feeling full or satiated.

THERMOGENICS

Thermogenic (fat-burning) pills help eliminate stubborn fat from the body. There are many thermogenic pills on the market, but the majority of them do not work.

Caffeine and ephedra are the only thermogenics that have been shown to produce moderate weight loss, although they have potentially adverse effects.[4]

Caffeine is available in pill form, but moderate daily coffee (one to four cups) or tea consumption is the ideal way to consume caffeine. A thermogenic effect is seen starting at 100 mg per day.[5][6][7]

Ephedra, known in Chinese as ma huang, has been scientifically proven time and again to effectively promote weight loss through its ability to increase thermogenesis and suppress appetite. However, ephedra has adverse effects—high blood pressure, tachycardia, central nervous system (CNS) excitation, and arrhythmia.

Bitter orange (Citrus aurantium) may be the best thermogenic substitute for ephedra. Research shows that those receiving a combination of bitter orange, caffeine, and St. John's wort lost weight.[8] Bitter orange increases resting metabolic rate and when taken for periods of up to 12 weeks, may result in modest weight loss.[9]

Chromium picolinate, Panax ginseng, green tea, garcinia cambogia extract (hydroxycitric acid), psyllium, green coffee extract, and St. John's wort may work for some people.[10][11][12][13][14][15][16][17]

Dr. Thomas Cowan, MD, who has helped numerous people lose weight in his holistic practice, recommends supplementing between meals with the fat-burning digestive enzyme lipase. He explains that taking lipase between meals three times per day as far away from food consumption as possible will often help mobilize fat stores. He recommends taking Chinese bitters two to three times per day to help clear out the fat breakdown products produced by the enzyme digestion.[18]

Raspberry ketone taken in high doses has been shown to prevent weight gain and promote the breakdown of fat.[19][20] Raspberry ketone is a natural phenolic compound of the red raspberry.

In one study, the combination of raspberry ketone, caffeine, capsaicin, garlic, ginger, and bitter orange promoted weight loss. Study participants who took this combination lost 7.8 percent of their fat mass, while the placebo group lost only 2.8 percent. (Both groups also reduced calories and exercised.)[21]

APPETITE SUPPRESSANTS

There is strong scientific support that dietary fiber intake prevents obesity. People who consume dietary fiber eat less and lose weight.[22][23] Fiber swells after ingestion and makes a person feel satiated.[24]

You can increase your consumption of dietary fiber with fruits, vegetables, whole grains, and legumes. You can also take a non-addictive fiber supplement such as apple pectin and oat bran available in pill or powder form. The powdered forms can be added to smoothies or to recipes for baked goods such as cookies, muffins, and pancakes.

In various studies, scientists found that Hoodia gordonii was an effective appetite suppressant.[25] [26] A Dutch anthropologist studying the primitive San Bushmen of the Kalahari Desert noticed that they ate the stems of the hoodia plant to suppress hunger during long hunting trips. The active ingredient in hoodia is the appetite-suppressing molecule P57. Scientists found that P57 acts on the brain in a manner similar to that of glucose. It tricks the brain into thinking that you are full even when you have not eaten. It also reduces interest in food and delays the time before hunger sets in.[27]

Guarana works in much the same way coffee does due to its high levels of caffeine. Caffeine suppresses the appetite. Guarana also improves memory, mood, and alertness. The lower dose of 75 milligrams produces more positive cognitive effects than higher doses do.[28]

DIABETES AND CHOLESTEROL

High cholesterol and diabetes are two of the most common conditions found among those who are overweight and obese.

High blood cholesterol is a major risk factor for heart and blood vessel disease. High cholesterol levels cause some cholesterol to deposit on the walls of the blood vessels. Over time, these deposits build up and become hard lumps (plaque). This causes the blood vessels to narrow, harden, and decrease blood flow which can lead to serious health risks such as hypertension, heart attack, or stroke.

There are two main types of cholesterol. Low-density lipoprotein (LDL) is known as "bad cholesterol," as it can clog the arteries. High-density lipoprotein (HDL) is the "good cholesterol," which transports some cholesterol back to the liver to be broken down. Doctors recommend that patients maintain lower LDL levels and higher HDL levels.

Diabetes is a disease in which the body is unable to properly use and store glucose (a form of sugar). Untreated, diabetes can lead to long-term complications such as heart attacks, strokes, blindness, kidney failure, blood vessel disease, nerve damage, and impotence in men.

High cholesterol and diabetes are life-threatening if not treated. Some people resort to pharmaceutical drugs to treat these conditions. However, pharmaceutical drugs typically have unpleasant and serious side effects. High cholesterol and diabetes can be treated naturally with minimal or no side effects.

Red rice extract has cholesterol-lowering properties. Some red rice extract preparations contain about 5 to 10 milligrams of lovastatin. These preparations may lower blood cholesterol levels, and work like statin drugs.[29]

Numerous studies have shown that omega-3 fish oil or oily fish consumed one or two times per week is beneficial for people with high cholesterol and diabetes. Fish oil lowers total cholesterol and very low-density lipoprotein (VLDL) and increases HDL.[30][31][32]

There are many medicinal herbs with strong anti-diabetic properties[33] that actually work better and have more diverse beneficial effects than do any pharmaceutical drugs presently available.

Gymnema sylvestre has been used in traditional Indian medicine for the treatment of diabetes for over 2,000 years. Gymnema came to be known as the "destroyer of sugar" because Ayurvedic physicians observed that chewing a few leaves suppressed the taste of sugar. ldResearch also shows that it prevents obesity. Gymnema reduces serum lipids, leptin, insulin, glucose, apolipoprotein B, and lactic acid dehydrogenase (LDH) levels while significantly increasing HDL cholesterol.[34]

Gymnema sylvestre targets several of the factors connected with diabetes, including chronic inflammation, obesity, enzymatic defects, and pancreatic cell function. No pharmaceutical drugs presently exert such a diverse range of effects. Researchers studying gymnema conclude that it may be useful for treating both insulin-dependent diabetes mellitus and non-insulin-dependent diabetes mellitus.[35]

Gymnema sylvestre in tea form offers the best results. A daily dose of 200 milligrams is optimal for weight management. The typical therapeutic dose for the treatment of hyperglycemia, standardized to contain 24 percent gymnemic acids, is 400 to 600 milligrams daily. Among adult-onset diabetics, ongoing use for periods of 18 to 24 months has been shown to be successful. In reducing the symptoms of glycosuria, the dried leaves are used in daily doses of three to four grams for three to four months. Gymnema extract acts gradually; therefore, it should be consumed regularly with meals for several months or years. It has no significant side effects when taken in proper doses.[36]

PHYTOCHEMICALS

Many of the health benefits of healthy foods have been attributed to their phytochemicals.[37] Phytochemicals are compounds that occur naturally in certain foods. "There are about 25,000 phytochemicals in the world, and we're finding that they perform special functions in the cells to help prevent diabetes, common forms of cancer, heart disease, age-related blindness and Alzheimer's disease," says David Heber, MD, PhD, director of the University of California, Los Angeles, Center for Human Nutrition and author of *What Color Is Your Diet?*

Scientists have discovered and isolated some of these phytochemicals to treat disease. For example, the anticancer drug paclitaxel is a phytochemical initially extracted and purified from the Pacific yew tree. However, research has shown that isolated phytochemicals do not have the same health benefits as do whole foods. An isolated phytochemical either loses its bioactivity or may not behave the same way as the compound in such whole foods as fruits, vegetables, whole grains, nuts, and seeds.[38]

One reason the French do not get fat despite a high-fat diet could be their moderate consumption of red wine, found to contain the phytochemical resveratrol. Resveratrol was shown to prevent weight gain despite a high-fat diet.[39]

Research shows that resveratrol affects energy metabolism and mitochondrial function and mimics the effects of calorie restriction. A randomized double-blind crossover study treated healthy, obese men with a placebo for 30 days and 150 milligrams per day of resveratrol for 30 days. Resveratrol decreased intrahepatic lipid content, circulating glucose, triglycerides, alanine-aminotransferase, and inflammation markers. The study demonstrated that 30 days of resveratrol supplementation induces metabolic changes in obese humans, mimicking the effects of calorie restriction.[40]

Curcumin is a phytochemical found in turmeric (Curcuma longa). It promotes weight loss and prevents obesity-related diseases.[41] Turmeric has been used for the treatment of diabetes in Ayurvedic and traditional Chinese medicine for centuries. Modern scientific research has found it to be effective for both the prevention and treatment of diabetes.[42] Turmeric has anti-inflammatory, antioxidant, anti-carcinogenic, anti-thrombotic, and cardiovascular protective effects.[43]

Curcumin has a poor oral bioavailability (a low percentage of what you consume is absorbed) and, thus, should be enhanced with other agents such as black pepper extract, called piperine.

Traditionally, chamomile tea and chamomile essential oil have been used to treat insomnia and to induce sedation (calming effects). Chamomile is widely regarded as a mild tranquilizer and sleep inducer. The nutrients and phytochemicals found in chamomile can help improve cardiovascular conditions, helps to manage diabetes, treat digestive disorders, stimulate the immune system, and provide protection against cancer.[44]

DAILY NUTRIENTS

Juicing of vegetables eliminates the fiber, leaving only the nutrients in a concentrated liquid. Eating 20 carrots every day would not typically be possible, but juicing 20 carrots a day makes it easy to consume a high level of nutrients. Invest in a high-quality masticating juicer, and juice a variety of vegetables every day. A masticating juicer eliminates the fiber from vegetables and leaves only the concentrated nutrients. You can juice apples, pears, pomegranates, kiwi fruit, carrots, broccoli, beets, kale, chard, collard greens, spinach, celery, cucumber, cabbage, parsley, arugula, dandelion greens, watercress, wheatgrass, and ginger.

Another effective way to nourish the body is to take ionic minerals. Ionic minerals are 1,000 times smaller than colloidal minerals.

Spirulina and chlorella are highly nutritious and rich sources of minerals.[45] Spirulina is about 51 percent to 71 percent protein, depending on its source. It is a complete protein containing all essential amino acids.[46][47] Spirulina has immunomodulation, anticancer, antiviral, and cholesterol reduction effects.[48]

Essential amino acids are not produced by the body and need to be taken in through diet or supplements. Vegans are especially at risk of developing an amino acid deficiency. The nine essential amino acids are histidine, isoleucine, leucine, lysine, methionine, phenylalanine, threonine, tryptophan, and valine.

Free-form amino acid supplements are a good way to ensure that all amino acids are provided to the body. Free-form amino acids don't require digestion. The term "free form" means the amino acids move quickly through the stomach and into the small intestine, where they're rapidly absorbed into the bloodstream.

Essential fatty acids (EFAs) are nutrients that humans need to obtain from food or supplements because the body cannot synthesize them.[49] Many illnesses are associated with a deficiency in omega-3 fatty acids.

Omega-3 is best obtained through wild salmon oil, cod liver oil, or krill oil. Flaxseed oil can be included in the diet, but is not the best source of EFAs. Research has found that the omega-3 fatty acids in fish oil "are more biologically potent than alpha-linolenic acid," or ALA, found in flaxseed, primrose, and borage oil. In other words, the body uses EPA and DHA from fish oil much more efficiently than it does omega-3 ALA from flaxseed, primrose, or borage.[50]

In one study, participants were given 15,000 milligrams of flaxseed oil (ALA) daily. At the end of 12 weeks not one of the participants had an increase of EPA or DHA within his or her blood plasma or red blood cells.[51]

Probiotics enhance the body's immune system[52] and may be useful for disease prevention and treatment, as well as the prevention of viral infections.[53] There are many strains of probiotic supplementation, but only certain colonizing probiotics strains like Bifidobacterium lactis HN019, Lactobacillus acidophilus L-14, and Lactobacillus plantarum Lp-115 have been well documented as adhering to human intestinal cells.[54]

CHAPTER SUMMARY

- Thermogenic (fat-burning) pills help promote fat loss and can be useful in eliminating stubborn fat from the body. Some scientifically proven effective thermogenics include bitter orange, caffeine, capsaicin, garlic, ginger, and raspberry ketone.

- The fat-burning digestive enzyme lipase taken three times per day between meals along with Chinese bitter may help mobilize fat stores.

- There is strong scientific evidence to support the theory that dietary fiber intake prevents obesity. People who consume dietary fiber eat less and lose weight. You can also take a non-addictive fiber supplement such as apple pectin and oat bran available in pill or powder form. The powdered forms can be added to smoothies or to recipes for baked goods such as cookies, muffins, and pancakes.

- Various studies have found that Hoodia gordonii is an effective appetite suppressant. Guarana is also effective in suppressing the appetite due to its caffeine content.

- High cholesterol can be treated naturally with red rice extract. Gymnema sylvestre in tea form has been found helpful for those with diabetes and obesity. A daily dose of 200 milligrams of gymnema sylvestre is optimal for weight management.

- The phytochemicals found in various foods help prevent disease and obesity. Resveratrol (found in red wine) was shown to prevent weight gain despite a high-fat diet. Curcumin is a phytochemical found in turmeric (Curcuma longa). It promotes weight loss and prevents obesity-related diseases such as diabetes and heart disease.

- To prevent nutritional deficiencies and maintain your overall health, include daily supplements in your diet. Such supplements include a whole food supplement, nano-ionic full-spectrum minerals, spirulina, chlorella, a free-form amino acid supplement, EFAs (wild salmon oil, cod-liver oil, or krill oil), and colonizing probiotics.

CHAPTER 5

HIDDEN FACTORS

If you find it impossible to control how much you eat, or if you encounter difficulty eating less frequently because you have a strong need to snack, you must address hidden health factors. In addition, if you have a severely stubborn weight-loss problem, underlying health problems are involved.

Rapid weight gain and an inability to lose weight could be caused by hypothyroidism, nutritional deficiencies, digestive problems, food intolerances, hormonal imbalance, stress, emotional problems, parasites, candida, toxins, insulin resistance, and leptin resistance.

TESTING FOR HIDDEN FACTORS

There are several tests you can use to determine your health status as well as discover hidden health factors hindering weight loss. These factors typically don't show up on standard tests.

Electrodermal screening (EDS), also called bioresonance therapy (BRT), is a fairly quick and effective health testing method. Electrodermal screening measures the electrical resistance on the skin's surface. The purpose is to detect energy imbalances along invisible lines of the body, called meridians. The screening can detect food sensitivities or allergies, nutritional deficiencies, organ stress, parasites, candida, heavy metals toxicity, and hormone imbalance.

Quantum biofeedback provides a comprehensive assessment of potential stressors such as viruses, parasites, nutritional deficiencies, allergies, and mental and emotional stress.

Live blood analysis (LBA) is the use of high-resolution dark-field microscopy to observe live blood cells. It provides information on the state of the immune system, nutritional deficiencies, oxygen deficiency, toxicity, pH imbalance, candida, parasites, and organ weakness.

Biological terrain assessment (BTA), also called quantitative fluid analysis (QFA), is an analysis of blood, urine, and saliva specimens that help detect fungi, pollutants, viruses, environmental poisons, and nutritional and oxygen deficiencies.

Applied kinesiology (AK) is a technique using the manual muscle test (MMT) as a diagnostic tool and for determining appropriate health treatments for an individual. There are many branches of applied kinesiology and considerable evidence exists testifying to the reliability and validity of manual muscle testing as a diagnostic tool.[1]

A medical intuition evaluation can provide information about current health status and also identify any mental and emotional factors that could be hindering weight loss. Many times, a medical intuitive can identify an imbalance within the body long before it manifests itself as disease. Some conventional medical doctors call on a medical intuitive for a second opinion.

Iridology analysis is a test conducted by a certified iridologist that examines the iris to determine current health status and future health issues. Iridology reveals constitutional strength, inherited strengths and weaknesses, toxicity levels, levels of inflammation, organ structure, and much more. The iridologist will make personalized recommendations for the improvement of health and prevention of disease.

Hair analysis is a screening test that identifies vitamin, mineral, and nutritional deficiencies as well as heavy metal toxicity. When new hair cells are forming in the hair follicle, they take in traces of substances going through the bloodstream of the individual.

The enzyme-linked immunosorbent assay (ELISA) test can accurately determine food allergies. Testing for food allergies is very important. Many people unknowingly consume foods that are harmful to their bodies.

The urine Indican test, also called an Obermeyer test, will determine digestive problems, malabsorption toxemia, and overgrowth of anaerobic bacteria.

Electrodermal screening is the most thorough and accurate type of screening. If you decide to test yourself for hidden health factors and can afford only one method, electrodermal screening is a good choice. Quantum biofeedback is also very accurate.

ELEVATED CORTISOL LEVELS

When you are under stress, whether physical (hard work, trauma, accident) or emotional (pain, anxiety, depression), it will be very difficult for you to lose weight.

Cortisol is a hormone that is released in response to stress and that tends to deposit fat around the waist; this is called visceral abdominal tissue. Visceral fat has been linked to an increase in both diabetes and heart disease. Visceral fat is accompanied by elevated triglycerides, reduced HDL cholesterol, elevated blood pressure, and/or elevated fasting plasma glucose.[2]

Cortisol tends to increase a person's appetite and cause that person to eat more than he or she normally would. Eating becomes a stress-relieving activity. After a while, eating in response to stress can become a learned habit.

Holy basil (Ocimum tenuiflorum) is an Indian herb that has been proven to reduce elevated cortisol levels.[3] In studies, holy basil has been shown to reduce stress, anxiety, depression, and exhaustion. It has anti-anxiety and anti-depressant properties, with effects comparable to diazepam and antidepressant drugs.[4] Holy basil is available as a tea or in capsules.

Low-intensity exercise is proven to reduce cortisol levels.[5] Pilates, yoga, meditation, qigong, tai chi, or a walk in a forest or along the beach are the most relaxing forms of exercise. Perform an activity you enjoy and make sure you feel refreshed and rejuvenated afterward—not exhausted. Exercising too hard and for too long can raise cortisol levels and actually increase stress.[6]

Make sure to get at least seven hours of sleep per night. Create a relaxing bedroom environment conducive to sleep. Lack of sleep elevates cortisol levels.[7]

Stress can deplete important nutrients such as B-complex, vitamin C, calcium, and magnesium. These nutrients are needed to balance the effects of stress hormones like cortisol. If these nutrients are depleted, resisting stress will become more difficult.

Stress increases the body's need for magnesium. Those under stress and who have a magnesium deficiency have an increased risk of hypertension, cerebrovascular and coronary constriction and occlusion, arrhythmia, and sudden cardiac death.[8]

When you are under stress, take a whole food supplement and eat plenty of foods high in magnesium, such as pumpkin seeds, squash seeds, sesame seeds, Brazil nuts, almonds, sunflower seeds, cashews, pine nuts, Swiss chard, spinach, prickly pear, and avocados.

The best way to test and monitor your stress levels is with heart rate variability (HRV) analysis. HRV is a powerful indicator of overall health. HRV analysis determines the probability of sudden, unexplained death by measuring minor variations in heart rate. HRV has become the standard test for measuring stress levels.

NUTRITIONAL DEFICIENCIES

One of the most ignored causes of weight gain is nutritional deficiencies. It is common to be overfed and undernourished. A lack of nutrients slows metabolism and reduces the body's ability to burn fat. Whether food is burned as energy or stored as fat is determined by a number of chemical reactions that take place in your body. These are activated by enzymes, which are, in turn, dependent upon vitamins and minerals. Therefore, if you are deficient in certain vitamins and minerals by even a small amount, you will gain weight. Deficiencies of nutrients can also trigger a ravenous appetite, uncontrollable cravings, the feeling of never feeling full after a meal, and hypothyroidism.

Food cravings and overeating can be signs of nutrient deficiency. Your body's desperate need for nutrients can cause you to overeat as the body attempts to get what it needs. If you eat foods with low nutritional value, you will gain weight and still feel hungry. A lack of chromium, sulfur or tryptophan can cause a craving for sweets.

You can survive for months or even years on poor-quality foods, but eventually it will catch up to you. Uncontrolled cravings can be an early sign of failing health.

Many people believe obesity is inherited and that there is nothing they can do about it. However, research has shown that magnesium and B complex help prevent obesity genes from expressing themselves. Experiments show that if a mouse with an obesity gene is deprived of B vitamins, the obesity will be expressed. However, if the mouse is fed plenty of B vitamins, it will remain thin. The process of metabolizing B vitamins is called methylation, and magnesium is necessary for this process.[9]

Magnesium and the B-complex vitamins activate enzymes that control digestion, absorption, and the utilization of proteins, fats, and carbohydrates. Lack of these necessary nutrients causes improper utilization of food, leading to hypoglycemia and obesity.

Magnesium deficiency has been shown to cause insulin resistance.[10] In their book, *The Magnesium Factor*, Mildred Seelig, MD, and Andrea Rosanoff, PhD, cite research showing that over half the insulin in the bloodstream is directed at the abdominal tissue. As more and more insulin is produced to deal with a high-sugar diet, abdominal fat increases to process the extra insulin.

Research shows that having low vitamin D levels can contribute to weight gain.[11] Vitamin D deficiency can lead to overeating. Lack of vitamin D disrupts communication from hormones responsible for sending signals to the brain indicating that you feel full.

Serotonin deficiency is associated with the brain's perception of starvation and hunger. When you have a shortage of serotonin in the brain, you will crave foods that help make serotonin, such as high-calorie, high GI carbohydrates. Research shows that 5-HTP effectively promotes weight loss in those with serotonin deficiency, as 5-HTP increases serotonin levels in the brain.[12]

Chromium deficiency is common in North America and can cause a strong craving for sweets. Supplementing with chromium picolinate is known to regulate blood sugar levels and reduce cravings for sweets.

The best way to correct nutritional deficiencies is by getting your nutritional needs from food. For example, Brazil nuts are extremely high in selenium, bananas are high in potassium, and sesame seeds are high in calcium and magnesium.

Rick Tague, MD, MPH, is a medical obesity specialist who recommends that everyone, regardless of age, take nutritional supplements daily.

Whole food supplements are made from concentrated whole foods. A whole food supplement is absorbed and assimilated by the body better than are synthetic supplements. Of course, besides taking a whole food supplement, consume an abundance of nutrient-rich foods to maintain optimum health for the long term. Make sure to get 7 to 10 daily servings of fruits and vegetables, nuts, seeds, fish, and legumes and beans. In addition, include superfoods in your diet. A superfood has extraordinarily high levels of vitamins, minerals, phytonutrients, and enzymes. Superfoods can be found in health food stores and include spirulina, raw cacao, chia seeds, hemp seeds, and wheatgrass juice.

BLOOD SUGAR AND INSULIN

A high-sugar diet and disruption of the circadian rhythm lead to an imbalanced blood sugar level.[13] An imbalanced blood sugar level reduces the body's ability to burn stored fat and causes weight gain. Too much glucose leads to high levels of blood sugar, which your body stores as fat.

Weight gain is a common side effect among people who take insulin therapy. When you take insulin, glucose is able to enter your cells and glucose levels in your blood drop. However, if you consume more calories than you need, your cells will get more glucose than they need. Glucose that your cells don't use accumulates as fat.

Insulin is the fat storage hormone and when your insulin levels rise, your body stops burning fat. It is impossible to burn body fat when insulin levels in the body are high. An insulin surge tells your body that plenty of energy is available and that it should stop burning fat and start storing it instead.

Research has shown that those who had low levels of insulin did not gain weight due to the fact that their fat cells burned more energy while storing less of it. The research indicates that people can maintain an ideal weight by increasing the time between their meals and by eliminating snacks (eating only one to three times per day).[14] Dr. James Johnson, an associate professor of cellular and physiological sciences, explains: "As crucial as insulin is for storing blood sugar, it can also be too much of a good thing. If we can maintain insulin levels at a happy medium, we could reverse the epidemic of obesity that is a risk factor for so many ailments—diabetes, heart disease, and cancer."

There are ways to limit insulin-associated weight gain, such as by eating foods low on the GI and using gymnema sylvestre.

Gymnema sylvestre has been found to repair and regenerate the pancreas and balance blood sugar levels.[15] Gymnema sylvestre is available in capsules or as a liquid tincture. Take gymnema sylvestre before each meal.

Eat foods that don't spike insulin levels sky high, such as high-fiber foods. When you eat refined grains, sugars, or carbohydrate-rich foods lacking fiber, the pancreas goes into overdrive to produce insulin.

FOOD SENSITIVITIES

Food allergies or food sensitivities can cause weight gain. "Food sensitivities are the common single cause of weight gain," says Dr. John Mansfield, author of *The Six Secrets of*

Successful Weight Loss. He has over 30 years of clinical practice and has helped hundreds of patients reach their ideal weights. "Food sensitivities were the prime cause in more than 70 percent of the patients I treated over a period of 31 years in clinical practice," says Dr. Mansfield.

"An estimated 60 to 80 percent of people are sensitive to one or more foods," says Ann Louise Gittleman, PhD, CNS.

A food intolerance generates the IgG immune response. It is an adverse reaction to a specific food, with symptoms such as irritable bowel syndrome (IBS), headaches, fatigue, eczema, migraine, fatigue, hives, and asthma. A food allergy generates the IgE immune response. The gold standard for diagnosing food intolerance is the double-blind placebo-controlled food challenge (DBPCFC).[16]

Another effective and accurate method of testing for food allergies and intolerance is EDS, also called BRT.

It's common to crave the foods to which we have an intolerance. According to Dr. Jonathan Brostoff, an allergy and environmental health expert, an estimated 50 percent of people with a food intolerance crave the very foods their bodies can't handle.

The most common allergens are cow's milk, chocolate, cola (the kola nut family), chicken eggs, soy, corn, peanuts, tree nuts, wheat, citrus fruits, tomatoes, fish, shellfish, artificial colors, food additives, and genetically modified crops.[17] [18 19]

A common symptom of food allergies or intolerances is headaches or migraines. You can use butterbur root extract to relieve migraines and headaches, but make sure to eliminate the foods that cause the headaches or migraines.

If you still want to consume the foods to which you are allergic or intolerant, you need to desensitize your body to them. Food allergies and food intolerances can be eliminated using a variety of methods. The Nambudripad's Allergy Elimination Technique (NAET) is a noninvasive, natural solution to eliminate allergies of all types. Allersodes are homeopathic preparations of highly diluted allergens used to desensitize the body to the allergen gradually. Annual desensitization may be necessary. Allersodes can be used along with methylsulfonylmethane (MSM) to reduce symptoms of allergies.[20] Start taking at least 6,000 milligrams of MSM per day for three weeks, then reduce to 3,000 milligrams per day.

Immunotherapy, consisting of sublingual immunotherapy (SLIT) or allergy injections, is an effective allergy treatment method.[21] It is similar to homeopathic allergy treatment. A small dose of an allergen is given under the tongue or through an injection, which reduces sensitivity to allergens.

TOXINS IN THE BODY

Toxicity of the body is a major cause of illness and weight gain. The WHO has acknowledged that environmental pollution is the underlying cause of nearly 80 percent of all chronic degenerative diseases.

There are tens of thousands of synthetic chemicals in the environment. Every year millions of pounds of chemical pollutants are released into the environment (and into our water and food). The body is designed to filter some of these toxins because it would not survive if it didn't. Health problems and weight gain occur when toxins are absorbed into the body faster than they can be eliminated. Toxins can damage the body's natural weight-control mechanisms.[22]

Body detoxification is a vital step toward preventing disease and losing weight. Just like the body must be regularly cleansed on the outside, the body must be regularly cleansed on the inside. American athlete Lee Haney said, "A systemic cleansing and detox is definitely the way to go. It is the key to fighting high blood pressure, heart disease, cancer, and other health-related illnesses."

Many naturopaths recommend daily cleansing of the body internally with warm water and lemon juice. Half a lemon or a full lemon is squeezed into a full glass of warm water and taken first thing in the morning on an empty stomach. Jethro Kloss, author of *Back to Eden*, said, "The medicinal value of the lemon is as follows: It is an antiseptic. It is also antiscorbutic, a term meaning a remedy which will prevent disease and assist in cleansing the system of impurities." Research has found that the consumption of lemon prevents body weight gain and body fat accumulation.[23]

Once a year, perform a complete internal body detox to thoroughly rid your body of toxins. Just remember that you will feel worse before you feel better. "The first couple of days on the detox diet aren't pleasant," said Carol Vorderman, a British media personality. During internal body cleansing, avoid pasteurized dairy products, meat, fried foods, sugar, artificial sweeteners, and table salt.

Once a year, perform a strict detox diet, eating no food and drinking only freshly squeezed lemon juice mixed with a tablespoon of maple syrup and a pinch of cayenne pepper for a period of seven days. One study found that this type of "lemon detox diet" reduced body fat and insulin resistance.[24]

You can perform a quick and simple full-body cleanse with quantum magnetization technology. Wu Qing Tong Ti Suite is a Chinese detoxification system that does the work of 100 cleanses in just 24 hours. Within 24 hours, a variety of brightly colored toxic substances are excreted from the body.

For those with very high levels of chemical contamination, a thoroughly deep internal cleanse can be conducted with the use of a far-infrared sauna. This is best done under the supervision of a medical professional familiar with this cleansing method. Heat from a far-infrared sauna stimulates the body to release toxins through sweating.

Silymarin is an antioxidant herb that protects the liver from toxins and also helps eliminate toxins from the liver. It can be taken daily in capsule form.

Many people have accumulated over 40 pounds of toxins in their colons, leading to enormously enlarged waistlines. Weight problems tend to start in the colon, then move on to other parts of the body.

Colon detoxification will flush out toxins from the colon and reduce the size of the waist. Colonics are effective for cleansing the colon. The colon can also be cleansed with the herbal combination of cape aloe leaf, rhubarb root, marshmallow root, and triphala churna. Non-addictive fiber supplements such as flax seeds and oat bran will keep the colon clean and can be taken daily. Make sure you are getting higher levels of fiber—between 30 grams to 60 grams per day.

POOR DIGESTION

Cravings for sugar, carbohydrates, and high-calorie foods indicate a high likelihood of digestive inflammation and poor digestion that is interfering with metabolism.

The complete digestive stool analysis (CDSA) is a test that provides an overview of digestion, absorption, intestinal function, and microbial flora. It also identifies pathogenic bacteria, parasites, and yeasts. You can have this test done to determine your digestive health status.

Gut microbiota, also called gut flora, are the "healthy bacteria" living in our intestines that are essential to good health and weight control. Gut microbiota helps the body digest certain foods that the stomach and small intestine have not been able to digest. They also help with the production of vitamins B and K, ensure proper digestive functioning, and help prevent obesity.

Many studies show that there is a difference in the composition of the gut microbiota of thin people and obese people. Obese people have higher levels of bad bacteria in their guts.[25] Anyone who has taken antibiotics is very likely to have a low level of "good bacteria" and a high level of "bad bacteria" in his or her gut.

Probiotics, in particular the bifidobacteria and especially bifidobacterium, are an important group of gut bacteria that controls the population of the bad bacteria in the gut. You can take a probiotic that contains bifidobacterium to increase your healthy levels of gut microbiota.

If you have food cravings you can take 2,000 to 3,000 milligrams of pine nut oil. Pine nut oil has been used in traditional folk medicine to treat ulcers and other digestive problems. It is effective in decreasing food cravings. Colostrum also helps heal an inflamed digestive tract.

Achlorhydria (no stomach acid) and hypochlohydria (low stomach acid) are very common digestive problems leading to poor nutrient absorption, food allergies, and parasite infections. A naturopath can perform a gastro-test to determine digestive function. Drinking one to two tablespoons of apple cider vinegar diluted in a glass of water before meals may increase hydrochloric acid (HCL) production.

It's helpful to realize that the stomach is not designed like a washing machine; rather, it stores ingested food in layers, one on top of another. To prevent digestive problems, it's best to follow the basic rules of "food combining."

Eat fruit and fruit juices on an empty stomach. Fruits leave the stomach within 20 to 40 minutes. Therefore, it is important to not eat them with any other foods, as doing so leads to fermentation, bloating, gas, and other digestive problems.

Eat soup at the beginning of a meal. The stomach processes and removes liquids before it attempts digestion of more solid food. Therefore, it's important to not drink large quantities of liquids before, during, and two hours after meals.

Cold drinks cause stomach cells to contract and prevent them from secreting the required amounts of digestive juices. Drink only hot water or hot drinks before, during, and after meals.

Contrary to popular belief, heartburn is not caused by too much stomach acid, but by too little of it. An insufficient supply of hydrochloric acid causes food to be undigested in the stomach for too long, producing stomach upset. Fresh ginger made into a hot tea with a pinch of cayenne pepper, or two tablespoons of organic apple cider vinegar in warm water taken 20 minutes before meals should help. If it doesn't, take betaine hydrochloride (HCl) capsules before meals.

CANDIDA OR PARASITES

Candida albicans overgrowth or a parasite infection can promote weight gain and make it difficult to lose weight by causing problems with the accumulation of fat, elevated blood levels of carbohydrates that do not respond normally to insulin, and systemic inflammation.[26]

Antibiotics, steroids, the birth control pill, and high sugar or carb consumption lead to an imbalanced overgrowth of candida albicans. Travel to foreign countries, drinking contaminated water, owning pets, or eating food prepared by others can lead to parasite infection. Electrodermal screening can accurately detect candida and parasites.

A common symptom of a Candida infestation is eating lots of sugar and carbs but still craving more. Parasite infection can be more subtle, but typical symptoms include diarrhea, stomach pain, gas, bloating, or fatigue.

Candida can be treated with olive leaf, berberine, and grapefruit seed extract. A "candida diet" is also helpful. The candida diet consists of eliminating sugar, carbohydrates, vinegar, mushrooms, cheese, peanuts, and high-sugar fruits for up to one year. For severe candida infection, take a low dose of nystatin along with oil of wild oregano (Origanum vulgare) and Two Feathers Healing Formula.

For parasite infection, take Two Feathers Healing Formula, an ancient American Indian herbal compound that is very effective at eliminating any type of parasite. Mild parasite infection responds well to the herbal combination of wormwood, wormseed, black walnuts, cloves, male fern, butternut, and orange peel.

HYPOTHYROID

The thyroid gland is an endocrine gland located in the lower front of the neck. The thyroid makes thyroid hormones, which are secreted into the blood and then carried to every tissue in the body. Thyroid hormone helps the body use energy, stay warm, and keep organs working as they should.

Hypothyroidism (underactive thyroid) causes weight gain and difficulty losing weight. Some people with low thyroid can have weight gain even when they severely restrict calories because of a very low basal metabolic rate. Treating hypothyroidism and thyroid dysfunction can help you lose weight.[27]

The diagnosis of hypothyroidism is usually made through measurements of Thyroid Stimulating Hormone (TSH) and Thyroxine (T4) levels found in blood tests. However, this method is ineffective at diagnosing cases of milder hypothyroidism (thyroid dysfunction). Laboratory blood test techniques give information about only the hormonal status of a patient at a particular point in time. The elevation of hormone levels in urine, however, assesses tissue exposure to thyroid hormones over a 24-hour period. The urine thyroid test can detect thyroid dysfunction that may otherwise go undetected in standard blood tests.

Hypothyroidism can be treated with the help of a naturopathic doctor and through such herbs as guggul, coleus (plectranthus barbatus), and bladderwrack.

According to Dr. Datis Kharrazian, 90 percent of people with hypothyroidism have Hashimoto's, an autoimmune hypothyroid condition in which the immune system attacks thyroid tissue.

It's commonly believed that hypothyroidism is due to insufficient iodine, but this isn't always the case, so check if you have iodine deficiency before supplementing with iodine. The best food sources of iodine are sea vegetables and seafood. Kelp or seaweed extract are the best supplemental sources of iodine.

HORMONAL LEVELS

Disruption of the circadian rhythm leads to hormonal imbalances of melatonin and serotonin. The increasing and decreasing levels of serotonin and melatonin indicate to the cells of the body whether it is night or day, and whether to be more active or less active.

The first essential step toward balancing melatonin and serotonin is getting enough sleep and following proper sleeping habits. Going to bed at no later than 10 p.m. is essential, as the deepest rest and most rejuvenation happen between 11 p.m. and midnight.

If you have a hard time falling asleep and have low energy during the day, take the supplement 5-HTP (5-Hydroxytryptophan) first thing in the morning and melatonin at night before bed. Melatonin is shown to reduce body weight and increase energy levels, as it improves sleep quality.[28]

5-HTP increases the production of serotonin and helps regulate sleep and appetite, as well as reduce food cravings. It is proven to decrease food intake and promote weight loss in those with serotonin deficiency.[29] Low levels of serotonin have been found to cause mood swings, depression, an inability to control food intake, and a craving for sweets and carbohydrates. Raising serotonin levels has been found to decrease depression and help control food intake.[30]

Imbalanced levels of the sex hormones estrogen and testosterone can promote weight gain in both men and women. Low testosterone levels and high estrogen levels in men can cause weight gain in older age. In women, high testosterone with lower estrogen and progesterone levels is a cause of weight gain during menopause.

Sex hormones can be tested using urine, serum, or saliva. Blood, saliva, and urine each have their own advantages. However, a 24-hour urine sample is most accurate because it is not susceptible to the hour-to-hour fluctuations seen in serum or salivary tests.

Long-term testosterone therapy in men with testosterone deficiency promotes permanent weight loss, reduced waist size, a lower BMI, and improved body composition.[31]

Menopause is also a high-risk time for weight gain in women. The average woman gains two to five pounds during menopausal transition; some women gain even more weight. There is typically a body fat distribution from peripheral to abdominal at menopause.

Natural hormone replacement therapy can help treat weight gain caused by a sex hormone imbalance. Herbs such as saw palmetto can be useful for lowering androgen levels. Pueraria mirifica has an estrogenic effect and is useful for perimenopausal women.[32]

Ghrelin and leptin are hormones that control appetite and regulate weight. Nearly all overweight and obese people have a problem with leptin resistance and have higher ghrelin levels.

Leptin is secreted primarily in fat cells and decreases hunger. Leptin tells the hypothalamus that you have enough fat, so you can eat less or stop eating. Ghrelin is secreted primarily in the lining of the stomach and increases hunger. Elevated ghrelin and leptin deficiency or leptin resistance make your brain think you are starving when that is not the case.[33][34]

Getting enough sleep (at least seven hours a night) is an important way to balance the hormones that control appetite. Research shows that those with reduced amounts of sleep had elevated ghrelin and reduced leptin levels, which leads to increased appetite and weight gain.[35]

To reverse leptin resistance and lower your ghrelin levels to reduce your appetite, practice proper meal timing and eat less frequently, which will reset your circadian rhythm. "In order to keep ghrelin low you need to eat on a schedule," explains Marjorie Nolan Cohn, a registered dietitian and certified personal trainer.

Try to eat as soon as possible upon rising in the morning, ideally within 30 minutes of waking. Eat a breakfast that has a lot of protein and fat. If you are hungry throughout the day, eat more protein in the morning.

Try to eat three meals a day initially. Then, work your way down to two meals a day. Eventually, as your hunger and cravings fade, you can adapt to eating only once a day.

Never snack between meals, initially and forever. Researcher Dr. Jack Kruse explains: "Snacking completely stresses the liver's metabolism and is just not recommended. Your liver needs to re-learn how to use gluconeogenesis normally again when you are asleep and awake. Snacking just destroys the timing and circadian clocks that work in unison with leptin."[36]

EMOTIONAL ISSUES

The emotional component to being overweight is huge, and it is largely ignored. As Adelle Davis, a nutrition pioneer, said, "To say that obesity is caused by merely consuming too many calories is like saying that the only cause of the American Revolution was the Boston Tea Party." Emotional issues can be the underlying reason for weight gain.

Research has found that traumatic life experiences during childhood and adolescence are common in overweight and obese people.[37] Traumatic life experiences lead to emotional stress. Emotional stress is a person's reaction to a situation that causes feelings of anxiety, fear, worry, tension, frustration, and anger. Emotional stress is difficult to measure because it is highly subjective. Every person responds differently to stressful events.

One study found that emotions like anger, depression and anxiety increase the risk of developing metabolic syndrome, a condition characterized by high triglyceride levels, elevated blood pressure, high blood sugar levels, low HDL cholesterol levels, and fat in the midsection.[38]

Emotional Armoring is a term used to describe suppressed emotional stress or emotional repression. Emotional repression is a coping mechanism our mind uses to handle situations we don't particularly want to deal with in the present moment. A common way in which we deal with unpleasant emotions is to suppress or ignore them. When you were teased, rejected, unloved, misunderstood, criticized, or mistreated, you felt hurt, pain, and anger. If the pain you felt was not acceptable or if you had no outlet for your feelings, your body suppressed your feelings. However, although negative emotions leave our conscious awareness, they aren't necessarily completely gone. Repressed emotional energy gets buried deep within the subconscious.

Emotional stress tends to cause emotional eating and cravings for sweet and fatty foods.[39] It has been shown that the more basic one's unfulfilled emotional needs, the more likely one is to engage in emotional eating.[40]

Unconsciously, a layer of fat on the body may serve to protect a person. Obesity is commonly protective sexually, physically, and socially. For example, in some cases, women who are victims of rape unconsciously gain weight in an effort to look unattractive and avoid another rape. More than half of the women Dr. Wendy Scinta treats in her medical weight-loss practice have sexual abuse in their past. Her treatment involves helping patients become comfortable with the attention that comes with a thinner body. "If there's obesity, there's a good chance, especially if there's morbid obesity, that something tragic happened in that person's history, at one point or another," she explains.

Vincent J. Felitti, MD, and colleagues have tracked more than 30,000 mostly middle-aged obese adults since 1982 and found that incest, rape, family suicide, and parental brutality were surprisingly common among overweight and obese people.[41] "We unexpectedly discovered that histories of childhood sexual abuse were common, as were histories of growing up in markedly dysfunctional households," the researchers explain. "The relationship between childhood sexual abuse and obesity later in life is major," says Dr. Felitti.[42]

Dr. Felitti found that people repeatedly fall into three categories: obesity is sexually protective; obesity is physically protective; or obesity is socially protective—people expect less from the obese person. "We slowly discovered that major weight loss is often sexually or physically threatening and that obesity, whatever its health risks, is protective emotionally," the researchers concluded.

Suzzanne Rosselot, who specializes in addictions, said, "If you grew up with trauma—emotional, sexual or physical—then you're going to respond by sort of developing some survival skills." That could mean unconsciously eating to put on weight as a way of becoming invisible (because society doesn't pay attention to fat people).

Jon Gabriel is a weight-loss expert who successfully lost more than 220 pounds (100 kilograms) without diets or surgery. He has helped many people lose weight without dieting by using only the mind-body approach. Gabriel explains that chronic weight gain is often caused by physical, emotional, or environmental triggers that confuse the body on a biological level. Therefore, if you are overweight, it is because your brain has a reason for it.

If you don't deal with the underlying issues, the weight will come back. It is very important to discover and treat any emotional issues. Those who are successful at losing weight but who don't treat the emotional issues behind their weight problems are very likely to regain the weight. A medical intuitive scan or quantum biofeedback will help determine underlying emotional issues.

Mindfulness-based stress reduction (MBSR) is an effective method of emotional stress reduction.[43] Research has found that mindfulness promotes significant weight loss.[44][45] Mindfulness can help those with emotional eating problems.[46]

The Healing Codes are a simple and powerful self-healing system and a form of energy medicine. The Healing Codes activate powerful healing centers that can allow the body to heal itself from emotional issues and stress.[47] You can search for a certified healing codes practitioner or learn the simple technique on your own.

There are many cases of people who have permanently lost weight without trying by using the Healing Codes or other emotional healing methods. Once underlying emotional issues are healed, people find themselves naturally drawn to healthier food choices and are less attracted to unhealthy foods.

Cognitive behavior therapy is helpful in treating anxiety or depression and in one study was found effective in producing long-term weight loss.[48]

LIFE FULFILLMENT

Some people eat out of boredom or depression related to a lack of fulfillment in their lives. If food served merely as sustenance, people would eat exactly what they needed and most would have no problem maintaining an ideal weight. However, food is also a great source of fulfillment and pleasure.

Psychologist Tom Griffiths states that there are plenty of people who never deal with emotional stress but simply eat for pleasure. "Food hits some of the same pleasure centers as antidepressants. Some of the neurotransmitters, such as serotonin and dopamine, are triggered by food. They are sources of pleasure," explains Griffiths.

Researchers have found that eating carbohydrate-rich foods releases into the brain the amino acid tryptophan, which then manufactures serotonin, a chemical that imparts feelings of calmness, peace, and well-being.[49]

To find fulfillment in life you need to develop a passion for something that will replace your passion for eating. Although there is nothing wrong with taking pleasure in a good meal, it's also important to find pleasure in simply living. Learn a new language, pursue a new hobby, make new friends, or do an activity that will keep you busy, stimulate you mentally, and help you find fulfillment in life.

CONCLUSION

Most people depend on their doctors to take care of their health. However, no one will care as much as you care; therefore, it's important to take charge of your own health and not depend entirely on someone else. Although you would like to attain a thin body naturally, weight problems could inspire you to take charge of your health and lead a longer, more productive life.

Anyone who wants to dramatically improve his or her health must start reading comprehensive health books that provide information about preventing and healing disease. The most comprehensive health and diet books are:

- *Timeless Secrets of Health and Rejuvenation* by Andreas Moritz

- *The Six Secrets of Successful Weight Loss* by Dr. John Mansfield

- *Nourishing Traditions: The Cookbook that Challenges Politically Correct Nutrition and the Diet Dictocrats* by Mary G. Enig and Sally Fallon

- *Nutrition and Physical Degeneration* by Weston A. Price

- *Mastering Leptin: Your Guide to Permanent Weight Loss and Optimum Health* by Mary Guignon Richards and Byron J. Richards

APPENDIX A: SUBSTITUTES

- Raw organic grass-fed goat's or sheep's milk and milk products; unsweetened rice, almond milk, or coconut milk instead of cow's milk

- Organic, grass-fed meat instead of conventional meat

- Organic, free-range eggs instead of conventional eggs

- Organic, gluten-free whole grains instead of grains with gluten

- Organic quinoa flour, almond flour, chickpea flour, buckwheat flour, or coconut flour instead of wheat flour

- Long-fermented organic "whole-milled" bread instead of wheat flour bread

- Organic apple cider vinegar instead of white vinegar

- Coconut palm sugar, stevia, raw Manuka honey instead of sugar or pasteurized honey

- Unrefined sea salt instead of table salt

- Grass-fed, organic high-vitamin butter oil or raw organic grass-fed goat's milk butter instead of butter or margarine

- Organic unrefined extra virgin coconut oil or ghee instead of vegetable oil for cooking

- Organic cold-pressed unrefined flaxseed or hempseed oil instead of vegetable oil for drizzling

- Carob bar instead of chocolate bar

- Vegetable chips (kale, sweet potato, butternut squash, or beet chips) instead of potato chips

APPENDIX B: OMAD DIET LIFESTYLE

PART I: PROPER EATING HABITS

- Eat only once per day, preferably in the morning or at lunchtime.

- If you are hungry, drink only homemade bone broth soup for dinner, but ideally, consume nothing at all.

PART 2: PROPER DIET (OPTIONAL)

BEVERAGES

- Bone broth soups from boiling bones of grass-fed cattle, bison, free-range poultry, or wild-caught fish

- Ultrapure water (reverse osmosis, distillation, ozonation, or ionic adsorption micron filter)

- Lacto-fermented drinks (water kefir, dairy kefir, Rejuvelac, kvass, kombucha tea)

- Healthy organic teas (herbal, white, green, oolong, yerba mate, rooibos)

- Organic coffee or coffee substitutes (Cafix, Dandy Blend)

PROTEIN

- 100-percent grass-fed meat from chicken, turkey, cow, lamb, duck, or wild game, or organ meat (heart, liver, brain, kidneys, tongue, tripe)

- Fresh shellfish in season, such as conch, oyster, lobster, shrimp, and crab

- Wild-caught fish and omega-3-rich fish such as mackerel, lake trout, herring, tuna, salmon, sardines, Atlantic sturgeon, lake whitefish, anchovies, bluefish, and sablefish

- Fish roe (fish eggs)

- Insects such as locusts, crickets, and grasshoppers, eaten fried, sautéed, boiled, or roasted

- Free-range, organic eggs from chickens, ducks, geese, quail, turkeys, ostriches, pheasants, and emu

FATS

- Grass-fed, organic deep yellow butter from cows, goats, or sheep

- Grass-fed, organic cream from goats or sheep

- Unrefined, cold-pressed flaxseed oil

- Cooking oil from organic extra virgin coconut oil, ghee, and animal fat (lard, beef, lamb, goose, duck)

DAIRY

- Unpasteurized, unhomogenized, grass-fed, organic, raw, whole milk and buttermilk from goats or sheep

- Grass-fed organic cottage cheese, Greek yogurt, kefir, plain yogurt, raw cheese

CARBOHYDRATES

- Organic whole grains prepared through soaking, fermenting, sprouting, and sour leavening

- Super fresh flour. After purchase, store your flour in the refrigerator. Better yet, grind your own flour out of whole grains with a grain grinder.

- Soaked and fermented pulses

- Long-fermented organic "whole-milled" bread (sourdough, whole wheat, rye, buckwheat, einkorn, emmer, kamut, spelt)

- Sprouted or soaked nuts and seeds

- Low GI tubers and vegetables

- Low GI fruits

CONDIMENTS

- Unrefined Celtic or Himalayan sea salt

- Apple cider vinegar

- Japanese rice vinegar (Kurosu)

- Super spices (peppers, turmeric, cinnamon, oregano, cumin, cayenne, cloves, parsley)

APPENDIX C: RESOURCES

RECOMMENED READING

Secrets from the Eating Lab: The Science of Weight Loss, the Myth of Willpower, and Why You Should Never Diet Again, by Traci Mann

Nourishing Traditions: The Cookbook that Challenges Politically Correct Nutrition and the Diet Dictocrats, by Mary G. Enig and Sally Fallon

The Fourfold Path to Healing, by Thomas Cowan

Eat Fat, Lose Fat, by Sally Fallon and Mary G. Enig

Timeless Secrets of Health and Rejuvenation, by Andreas Moritz

RECOMMENDED WEBSITES

The Weston A. Price Foundation
www.westonaprice.org

Body Building
www.bodybuilding.com

Natural Database
www.naturaldatabase.com

RECOMMENDED MAGAZINES

FitnessRX for Women
www.fitnessrxwomen.com

FitnessRX for Men
www.fitnessrxformen.com

FOOD SOURCES

Grass-fed, organic meat, dairy, and eggs
www.eatwild.com
www.uddermilk.com

Healthy desserts
www.wellnessbakeries.com
www.justdeliciousbakery.com

HEALTH TESTS

Genova Diagnostics
www.gdx.net

Rocky Mountain Analytical
www.rmalab.com

Doctor's Data
www.doctorsdata.com

Life Technologies
www.lifetechnologies.com

NeuroScience
www.neurorelief.com

Counsyl
www.counsyl.com

APPENDIX D: MEAL PLANS

The following meal plans and recipes are based on the Weston Price diet and the Mediterranean diet, as well as on the principles of Ayurveda, the Satiety Index, the GI, and GL. All the recipes for the italicized dishes mentioned in the two meal plans are found in Appendix E.

If you are following the one meal per day plan, select a time that is most convenient for you to eat that one meal per day, whether it be breakfast or lunch. Remember that when eating one meal per day, it's important to feel satisfied and full and that there is no strict portion sizes except wise moderation.

THE ONE MEAL PER DAY MEAL PLAN

DAY 1
Morning
Two glasses of filtered warm or hot water with the freshly squeezed juice of half a lemon or lime
During the day
Drink *Hot Ionized Water*

Full-course meal

Starter: *Raw Milk Tonic*

First course: *Quinoa Salad*

Main course: Grass-fed steak with a side of organic vegetables sautéed in coconut oil and a pinch of turmeric; a sprinkle of Himalayan or Celtic sea salt to taste

Dessert: A handful of unsalted, unroasted organic nuts of your choice, or any dessert of your choice that has been sweetened with a natural, low GI sweetener

Beverage: Gymnema tea

DAY 2
Morning
Two glasses of filtered warm or hot water with the freshly squeezed juice of half a lemon or lime

During the day
Drink *Hot Ionized Water*

Full-course meal
Starter: *Chicken Bone Broth*

First course: *Tabbouleh Salad*

Main course: 1 organic free-range chicken leg or thigh with boiled organic potatoes; a sprinkle of Himalayan or Celtic sea salt to taste

Dessert: ½ cup of organic grass-fed cottage cheese drizzled with raw honey or any dessert of your choice (sweetened with a natural, low GI sweetener)

Beverage: Gymnema tea

DAY 3
Morning
Two glasses of filtered warm or hot water with the freshly squeezed juice of half a lemon or lime

During the day
Drink *Hot Ionized Water*

Full-course meal
Starter: *Butternut Squash Soup*

First course: *Sauerkraut Salad*

Main course: *Grilled Chicken with Chili and Sesame Seeds*

Dessert: *Coconut Milk Ice Cream*

Beverage: Gymnema tea

DAY 4
Morning
Two glasses of filtered warm or hot water with the freshly squeezed juice of half a lemon or lime

During the day

Drink *Hot Ionized Water*

Full-course meal
Starter: *Oxtail Broth*

First course: *Cranberry Feta Salad*

Main course: *Maple Salmon* topped with a teaspoon of grass-fed butter and a side of quinoa or brown rice (soaked overnight); a sprinkle of Himalayan or Celtic sea salt to taste

Dessert: *Macaroons* or a dessert of your choice

Beverage: Gymnema tea and a cup or two of a lacto-fermented drink of your choice (rejuvelac, kvass, kefir, or kombucha tea)

DAY 5
Morning
Two glasses of filtered warm or hot water with the freshly squeezed juice of half a lemon or lime

During the day
Drink *Hot Ionized Water*

Full-course meal
Starter: *Mediterranean Vegetable Soup* with a slice of long-fermented organic "whole-milled" bread

First course: *Seaweed Salad*

Main course: Bison steak and *Oven-roasted Vegetables*

Dessert: *Almond Cake*

Beverage: Gymnema tea

DAY 6
Morning
Two glasses of filtered warm or hot water with the freshly
squeezed juice of half a lemon or lime

During the day
Drink *Hot Ionized Water*

Full-course meal
Starter: *Coconut Milk Soup*

First course: *Fruit Salad*

Main course: *Greek Lamb Chops*

Dessert: *Healthier Chocolate Cake*

Beverage: Gymnema tea and a cup or two of a lacto-
fermented drink of your choice (rejuvelac, kvass, kefir, or
kombucha tea)

DAY 7
Morning
Two glasses of filtered warm or hot water with the freshly
squeezed juice of half a lemon or lime

During the day
Drink *Hot Ionized Water*

Full-course meal
Starter: *Lentil Soup* with a slice of long-fermented organic "whole-milled" bread

First course: *Mediterranean Salad*

Main course: A bowl of regular oatmeal (not quick-cook instant oats, as they have a GI of 66, while regular oats have a GI of 55) with goat or sheep's milk, sprinkled with flaxseed, chia seeds, almonds, walnuts, goji berries, açai berries, gooseberries, and a sprinkle of ground cinnamon

Dessert: *Chocolate Chip Cookie*

Beverage: Gymnema tea and a cup of grass-fed, organic buttermilk

DAY 8
Morning
Two glasses of filtered warm or hot water with the freshly squeezed juice of half a lemon or lime

During the day
Drink *Hot Ionized Water*

Full-course meal
Starter: *Mediterranean Cold Yogurt Soup*

First course: *Tuna Salmon Salad*

Main course: *Quesadillas* with a side of *Baked Beans*

Dessert: *Whole-Grain Pancakes* drizzled with pure organic Canadian maple syrup

Beverage: Gymnema tea and a cup of unpasteurized, unhomogenized, grass-fed, organic, raw, whole milk from a goat or sheep

THE TWO MEALS PER DAY PLAN

DAY 1
Breakfast: Gymnema tea, one glass of filtered warm or hot water with the freshly squeezed juice of half a lemon, and *Raw Milk Tonic*

Lunch: *Quinoa Salad, Maple Salmon,* and *Seaweed Salad.*

During the day: Drink *Hot Ionized Water*

Dinner (optional): Bone broth soup

DAY 2
Breakfast: Gymnema tea, a cup or two of grass-fed, organic buttermilk and *Scrambled Eggs*; a sprinkle of Himalayan or Celtic sea salt to taste

Lunch: *Lentil Soup* and *Tuna Salmon Salad*

During the day: Drink *Hot Ionized Water*

Dinner (optional): Bone broth soup

DAY 3
Breakfast: Gymnema tea, one glass of filtered warm or hot water with the freshly squeezed juice of half a lemon, and *Amaranth with Walnuts and Honey*

Lunch: Mackerel pan-seared in organic extra virgin coconut oil and *Amaranth Salad*

During the day: Drink *Hot Ionized Water*

Dinner (optional): Bone broth soup

DAY 4

Morning: Gymnema tea and a cup or two of a lacto-fermented drink of your choice (rejuvelac, kvass, kefir, or kombucha tea)

Lunch: Bison steak and *Oven-roasted Vegetables*

During the day: Drink *Hot Ionized Water*

Dinner (optional): Bone broth soup

DAY 5

Breakfast: Gymnema tea and a cup or two of unpasteurized, unhomogenized, grass-fed, organic, raw, whole milk from a goat or sheep

Lunch: Grass-fed beef and *Potato Salad*

During the day: Drink *Hot Ionized Water*

Dinner (optional): Bone broth soup

DAY 6

Breakfast: Gymnema tea, one glass of freshly squeezed grapefruit juice and *5-Grain Energy Porridge*

Lunch: Grass-fed lamb and organic vegetables sautéed in organic extra virgin coconut oil

During the day: Drink *Hot Ionized Water*

Dinner (optional): Bone broth soup

DAY 7

Breakfast: Gymnema tea and a bowl of regular oatmeal (not quick cook instant oats since they have a GI of 66, while regular oats have a GI of 55) with goat's or sheep's milk, sprinkled with flaxseed, chia seeds, almonds, walnuts, goji berries, açai berries, gooseberries and a sprinkle of ground cinnamon.

Lunch: Lake trout pan-seared in organic extra virgin coconut oil and *Wild Rice Salad*

During the day: Drink *Hot Ionized Water*

Dinner (optional): Bone broth soup

DAY 8

Breakfast: Gymnema tea and a bowl of regular oatmeal (not quick cook instant oats since they have a GI of 66, while regular oats have a GI of 55) with goat's or sheep's milk, sprinkled with flaxseed, chia seeds, almonds, walnuts, goji berries, açai berries, gooseberries and a sprinkle of ground cinnamon.

Lunch: *Mediterranean Cold Yogurt Soup*, *Tuna Salmon Salad*, and *Quesadillas*

During the day: Drink *Hot Ionized Water*

Dinner (optional): Bone broth soup

APPENDIX E: RECIPES

HOT IONIZED WATER

Ingredients:
Pure filtered water (reverse osmosis, distillation, ozonation, or ionic adsorption micron filter)

Directions:
1. Boil about 20 to 24 ounces of pure filtered water for 15 to 20 minutes.

2. Immediately pour the boiled water into a Thermos; stainless steel is fine. In the Thermos, the water will stay ionized for up to 12 hours or for as long as it remains hot.

3. Take 1 or 2 sips every half hour all day long, and drink it as hot as you would sip tea. In addition, drink regular, cold, or room-temperature water when you are thirsty.

Note: You can drink hot ionized water for a certain duration, such as every day for three to four weeks or ongoing. This specially prepared water should not substitute for normal drinking water. It doesn't hydrate the cells like normal water does; the body uses it only to cleanse the tissues.

BONE BROTH

Ingredients:
4 pounds organic, grass-fed, cut-up meat bones of beef, lamb, bison, or venison
20 cups filtered water
¼ cup organic apple cider vinegar
3 cups organic onions, coarsely chopped
4 cups organic carrots, coarsely chopped
3 cups organic celery sticks, coarsely chopped
2 teaspoons Celtic or Himalayan sea salt to taste (after broth is finished cooking)

Directions:
1. Place the meat bones on a large cookie sheet or roasting pan and brown them in the oven at 350°F for 45 minutes.

2. Remove the bones from the oven. After the bones cool, pop out the marrow and meaty bits with a knife. Place the bits in a mason jar to be used in gravies and puréed soups.

3. Place the bones in a stockpot; add the water, apple cider vinegar, and vegetables. Deglaze your roasting pan with hot water and get up all of the brown bits. Pour this liquid into the pot. Do not skip adding the vinegar, as it draws the minerals out of the bones and adds a nice flavor to the soup. If you are sensitive to apple cider vinegar, use lemon juice instead.

4. Bring the ingredients to a boil and remove the scum that rises to the top. Don't worry about removing the floating fat.

5. Reduce the heat to its lowest point, cover, and simmer for at least 12 hours and as long as 48 hours. The longer you cook the stock, the more flavorful and nutritious the broth will be.

6. Strain the stock through a stainless steel strainer into a large bowl, then pour the broth into wide-mouth mason jars. Let the jars sit until they are just warm to the touch, then freeze or refrigerate. The remaining fat layer preserves the broth and helps keep out microbes.

CHICKEN BONE BROTH

Ingredients:
1 whole organic chicken carcass (bones from a roast chicken dinner)
12 cups filtered water
1 cup organic onion
4 cups organic vegetables (carrots, celery leaves)
½ cup organic apple cider vinegar
Seasoning (parsley and basil stems)
1 teaspoon Celtic or Himalayan sea salt to taste (after broth is finished cooking)

Directions:
1. Strip the chicken and save the meat in a container to use in the soup later. Put all the ingredients into a large pot and bring to a boil.

2. Reduce heat to its lowest point, cover, and simmer. Cook for 8 to 12 hours. You can cook this for up to 24 hours if you own a Crock-Pot.

OXTAIL BROTH

Ingredients:
4 pounds organic, grass-fed oxtails
¼ cup organic apple cider vinegar
2 organic carrots, coarsely chopped
1 organic onion, coarsely chopped
3 sticks organic celery, coarsely chopped
3 teaspoons dried herbs

Directions:
1. Place oxtails in a large flameproof baking pan and bake at 400° until browned.

2. Place in a Crock-Pot with the remaining ingredients. Place the baking pan over a burner and add filtered water to the pan.

3. Bring to a boil and stir, scraping up all the residue in the pan. Add this water to the Crock-Pot along with enough water to cover the bones. Bring to a simmer and skim off any scum that rises to the top.

4. Cover and simmer for about 12 hours.

5. Let the broth cool, remove the bones and vegetables with a slotted spoon, and strain the broth into a bowl. Chill and remove any fat that comes to the top.

6. Transfer to containers and store in the refrigerator if you plan on using the broth within three days. For long-term storage, store in the freezer. You can use this broth in nourishing soups, stews, and sauces, or drink it like tea.

COCONUT MILK SOUP

Ingredients:

4 cups homemade chicken broth

1 cup whole organic coconut milk

1-inch piece fresh organic ginger, peeled and chopped

1 teaspoon Celtic or Himalayan sea salt

Juice of 1 organic lemon or 2 limes

¼ teaspoon red pepper flakes

Directions:

1. Place all ingredients in a pot and whisk together.

2. Simmer for about 10 minutes.

Serves 4 to 6.

BUTTERNUT SQUASH SOUP

Ingredients:
2 tablespoons organic extra virgin coconut oil
1 organic carrot, diced
1 organic celery stalk, diced
1 organic onion, diced
4 cups cubed organic butternut squash, fresh or frozen
½ teaspoon chopped fresh thyme
4 cups organic chicken broth
½ teaspoon Celtic or Himalayan sea salt
½ teaspoon ground black pepper

Directions:
1. Heat the coconut oil in a large soup pot. Add the carrot, celery, and onion. Cook until the vegetables have begun to soften and the onion turns translucent, 3 to 4 minutes.

2. Stir in butternut squash, thyme, chicken broth, salt, and pepper. Bring to a boil, reduce heat, and simmer until squash is fork-tender, about 30 minutes.

3. Use an immersion blender to purée the soup. Alternatively, let the soup cool slightly and carefully purée in batches in an upright blender.

Serves 6.

CARROT SQUASH SOUP

Ingredients:
2 pounds organic butternut squash, peeled and cubed
3 cups organic carrots, peeled and cubed
2 cloves garlic, crushed
1-inch cinnamon stick
1 teaspoon ground coriander
½ teaspoon nutmeg
2 bay leaves
1 cup rice milk
1 tablespoon organic cashew or almond butter

Directions:
1. Place the butternut squash, carrots, onion, garlic, and parsley root in a pot with enough water to cover. Bring to a boil, add spices (cinnamon stick, coriander, nutmeg, bay leaves), and reduce heat to a simmer. Skim off and discard any foam that forms on the top. Simmer until vegetables are tender.

2. Discard the bay leaves and cinnamon stick. Process the cooked vegetables in a blender or food processor, and add cashew or almond butter.

3. When the soup is blended, thin the soup with rice milk if necessary.

Serves 4.

LENTIL SOUP

Ingredients:
1 cup organic lentils, soaked in warm water for about 7 hours
4 tablespoons grass-fed butter
2 large organic onions, chopped
Juice of 2 organic lemons
4 large organic carrots, chopped
1 teaspoon Celtic or Himalayan sea salt
4 tablespoons curry powder
1 cup grass-fed cream or sour cream
3 cups chicken broth or water

Directions:
1. In a large pot, cook the carrots and onion in butter over low heat until the vegetables are soft. Stir in curry powder and salt. Drain the lentils and add to the pot along with the chicken stock or water.

2. Bring to a slow boil and cook until the lentils are soft, about 30 minutes.

3. Blend the soup with a handheld blender until smooth. Stir in the cream and lemon juice. If the soup is too thick, add more water or broth.

Serves 6.

BLACK BEAN SOUP

Ingredients:
1 tablespoon organic extra virgin coconut oil
1 small organic onion, chopped
1 tablespoon chili powder
1 teaspoon ground cumin
2 15-ounce cans organic black beans
3 cups filtered water
½ cup homemade salsa
¼ teaspoon Celtic or Himalayan sea salt
1 tablespoon lime juice
4 tablespoons grass-fed sour cream
2 tablespoons organic cilantro, chopped

Instructions:
1. Heat the coconut oil in a large saucepan over medium heat. Add onion and cook, stirring, until they begin to soften, 2 to 3 minutes.

2. Add chili powder and cumin and cook, stirring, for about 1 minute.

3. Add beans, water, salsa, and salt. Bring to a boil; reduce heat and simmer for 10 minutes. Remove from heat and stir in lime juice.

4. Transfer half the soup to a blender and puree. Stir the puree back into the saucepan. Serve garnished with sour cream and cilantro.

Serves 4 to 6.

MEDITERRANEAN VEGETABLE SOUP

Ingredients:
1 tablespoon organic extra virgin olive oil
1 organic onion, diced
1 organic carrot, halved lengthwise and sliced
2 stalks organic celery, sliced
3 cloves organic garlic, minced
2 cups free-range organic chicken or beef broth
2 cups filtered water
1 can (14½ ounces) diced organic tomatoes, not drained
1 tablespoon fresh organic basil, chopped
¼ teaspoon organic oregano
Celtic or Himalayan sea salt and pepper, to taste
1 15-ounce can cannellini or white beans, drained and rinsed
1 cup whole wheat pasta bows (or brown rice pasta)

Directions:
1. Heat the oil in a heavy saucepan over medium heat. Add the onion, carrot, and celery, and sauté until tender, about 5 minutes. Add the garlic, broth, water, tomatoes, basil, oregano, salt, pepper, and beans.

2. Bring to a boil, reduce heat, and simmer for 10 minutes.

3. Add the pasta bows and cook 10 to 15 minutes, stirring occasionally until the pasta is cooked.

Serves 4 to 6.

MEDITERRANEAN YOGURT SOUP

Ingredients:
2 pounds organic goat yogurt, made from whole milk
1 pint grass-fed heavy cream
1 tablespoon Celtic or Himalayan sea salt
2 tablespoons organic lemon juice
2 tablespoons organic garlic cloves, minced
8 tablespoons organic feta cheese, crumbled
4 tablespoons organic olives, Kalamata (pits removed and cut into pieces)
½ cup organic bell pepper
8 tablespoons organic spring onions, chopped
8 tablespoons organic pistachio nuts, shells removed and ground up coarsely

Directions:
1. For each serving put ½ cup of yogurt in a bowl, then add 1/8 to ¼ cup cold water (depending on the thickness desired), 1/8 cup cream, 1 teaspoon salt, 1 tablespoon lemon juice, and 1 teaspoon minced garlic, and blend until creamy smooth.

2. Add to each individual bowl 2 tablespoons feta cheese, 1 tablespoon olives, 2 to 3 tablespoons bell peppers, and 2 tablespoons spring onions, and mix. Sprinkle 2 tablespoons of ground pistachio nuts on top. Chill prior to serving.

Note: This soup is best when using whole creamy milk yogurt, which can be found in Greek and Middle Eastern grocery stores (or use homemade yogurt).

Serves 4.

RAW MILK TONIC

Ingredients:
2 cups whole organic, raw milk
2 raw free-range egg yolks
2 tablespoons organic maple syrup
¼ teaspoon vanilla extract

Directions:
1. Use a whisk to blend the egg yolks into the milk.

2. Stir in the maple syrup and vanilla extract and serve immediately.

Serves 1 or 2.

COCONUT BANANA BREAD

Ingredients:
4 large free-range eggs, lightly beaten
4 ripe organic bananas, mashed (2 cups)
3 tablespoons organic maple syrup
2 teaspoons vanilla extract
½ cup organic coconut flour
1 teaspoon Celtic or Himalayan sea salt
2 teaspoons ground organic cinnamon
1 teaspoon organic baking powder
½ teaspoon organic baking soda

Directions:
1. Preheat the oven to 375°F. Lightly oil an 8-inch by 5-inch loaf pan.

2. In a mixing bowl, combine the mashed banana, beaten eggs, maple syrup, and vanilla extract.

3. In a separate bowl, stir together the coconut flour, salt, cinnamon, baking powder, and baking soda.

4. Pour the dry mixture into the bowl with the wet mixture and stir until combined. Allow batter to sit for 5 minutes before pouring it into the prepared loaf pan. Bake on the center rack in the oven for 45 to 55 minutes, until the loaf tests clean.

5. Remove bread from the oven and allow it to sit for 30 minutes before turning it out onto a cutting board. Cut thick slices and serve with grass-fed butter and organic raw honey.

Yields 1 loaf of bread

QUESADILLAS

Ingredients:
4 organic whole-grain flour tortillas
2 cups grated organic cheese
1 cup organic meat or sausage, chopped
1 small organic onion, peeled and chopped
1 small organic green jalapeno pepper, seeded and chopped fine
½ cup organic lard
Grass-fed sour cream
1 organic avocado, peeled and cut into wedges

Directions:
1. Melt the lard in a large cast iron skillet. Place one tortilla in the pan. Place ½ cup cheese, ¼ cup of the optional chopped meat or sausage, and ¼ cup of the onion and peppers on half the tortilla and fold the other half over to cover the cheese. Repeat the process in the remaining pan space so that you are cooking two quesadillas at the same time.

2. When the underside is brown, turn over and brown the remaining side.

3. Place on a platter in a warm oven while preparing the other two quesadillas. Serve with sour cream and wedges of ripe avocado.

Serves 4.

OVEN-ROASTED VEGETABLES

Ingredients:

2 organic sweet potatoes, cubed

3 organic new potatoes, cubed

1 organic red onion, quartered and pieces separated

2 organic zucchini, sliced 1 inch thick

2 organic summer squash, sliced 1 inch thick

1 (8-ounce) bag organic baby carrots

8 ounces organic button mushrooms, ends of stems cut off

1 tablespoon fresh organic thyme, chopped (1 teaspoon dried)

2 tablespoons fresh organic rosemary, chopped (2 tablespoons dried)

1 teaspoon dried basil (optional)

3 teaspoons garlic, minced

¼ cup organic extra virgin olive oil

2 tablespoons organic balsamic vinegar

Organic extra virgin coconut oil cooking spray

Celtic or Himalayan sea salt and pepper, to taste

Directions:

1. Preheat oven to 450°F.

2. Chop all the vegetables, as specified in the ingredient list.

3. Mix thyme, rosemary, basil, garlic, olive oil, balsamic vinegar, salt, and pepper in a bowl; set aside.

4. Put the chopped vegetables in a large bowl, then pour the oil/vinegar/herb mixture over the vegetables. Stir until all the vegetables are coated evenly.

5. Spray a baking sheet or roasting pan tray with organic extra virgin coconut oil cooking spray.

6. Spread the vegetables evenly on the pan and pour the remaining oil/vinegar/herb mixture on top.

7. Roast for 40 minutes, stirring every 15 to 20 minutes or until potatoes are soft when poked with a fork.

CRANBERRY FETA SALAD

Ingredients:
2 cups mixed organic salad greens (Leaf lettuce, endive, radicchio)
1 cup dried organic cranberries
4 ounces crumbled grass-fed feta cheese
½ cup organic walnuts
2 tablespoons organic balsamic vinegar
1 tablespoon raw organic honey
1 teaspoon organic Dijon mustard
¼ teaspoon ground black pepper
¼ cup organic extra virgin olive oil

Directions:
1. Toss greens, cranberries, cheese, and walnuts in a large bowl.

2. Mix vinegar, honey, mustard, and pepper with a wire whisk until well blended.

3. Gradually add oil, whisking constantly until well blended. Pour over salad; toss to coat. Serve immediately.

Serves 4.

SAUERKRAUT SALAD

Ingredients:

1-quart organic sauerkraut, drained
1 organic onion, chopped
2 stalks organic celery, chopped
1 organic bell pepper, chopped
1 large organic carrot, chopped
1 (4-ounce) organic pimento pepper, drained and diced
1 teaspoon organic mustard seed
1½ cups coconut palm sugar
1 cup organic extra virgin olive oil
½ cup apple cider vinegar

Directions:

1. In a large bowl, mix together sauerkraut, onion, celery, green bell pepper, carrot, pimientos, and mustard seed.

2. In a small saucepan, mix together coconut palm sugar, olive oil, and apple cider vinegar. Bring to a boil. Remove from heat.

3. Pour sugar mixture over salad, cover, and leave it in the refrigerator for 2 days before serving to allow the flavors to develop.

Serves 6.

QUINOA SALAD

Ingredients:
6 cups organic baby spinach
2 cups organic cucumbers, diced
1 organic avocado, halved, seeded, peeled, and diced
1 cup cooked organic quinoa
¼ cup almonds, walnuts, and pecan halves
¼ cup crumbled organic goat cheese

Balsamic vinaigrette:
¼ cup organic extra virgin olive oil
¼ cup organic balsamic vinegar
2 cloves organic garlic, pressed
1 teaspoon rapadura or granulated maple sugar

Directions:
1. Place spinach cucumbers, avocado, quinoa, pecans, and goat cheese in a large bowl.

2. To make the vinaigrette, whisk together olive oil, balsamic vinegar, garlic, and sugar in a small bowl.

3. Pour dressing on top of the salad and gently toss to combine. Serve immediately.

Serves 6.

TABBOULEH SALAD

Ingredients:

½ cup fine organic bulgur

3 tablespoons organic extra virgin coconut oil

1 cup boiling-hot water

2 cups finely chopped fresh flat-leaf organic parsley

½ cup finely chopped fresh mint

2 medium organic tomatoes, cut into ¼-inch pieces

½ seedless European cucumber, peeled, cored, and cut into ¼-inch pieces

3 tablespoons fresh organic lemon juice

¾ teaspoon Celtic or Himalayan sea salt

¼ teaspoon black pepper

Directions:

1. Stir together bulgur and 1 tablespoon oil in a heatproof bowl. Pour boiling water over, then tightly cover the bowl with plastic wrap and let stand 15 minutes. Drain in a sieve, pressing on bulgur to remove excess liquid.

2. Transfer bulgur to a bowl and toss with remaining ingredients, including 2 tablespoons oil, until combined well.

Serves 4 to 6.

POTATO SALAD

Ingredients:

2 pounds (907 grams) small organic yellow, red, or white potatoes

1 tablespoon organic apple cider vinegar

½ cup grass-fed sour cream

¼ cup organic mayonnaise (preferably homemade)

1 tablespoon organic yellow mustard

½ cup red onion, finely chopped

½ cup organic celery, finely chopped

1/3 cup organic dill pickles, finely chopped

2 hard-boiled free-range eggs, peeled and chopped

¼ cup fresh herbs, chopped

Celtic or Himalayan sea salt and freshly ground black pepper, to taste

Directions:

1. Add potatoes to a large pot, then cover with 1½ inches of water. Bring water to a boil, then reduce to a low simmer. Cook 15 to 20 minutes or until potatoes can easily be pierced with a fork.

2. While potatoes cook, set up an ice bath. Add cold water to a medium bowl, then add ice. Drain potatoes, then add to ice bath. Once cooled, peel potatoes by gently pinching the skin and pulling it away.

3. Chop peeled potatoes into bite-size chunks, then add to a large bowl. Scatter 1 tablespoon of vinegar over potatoes and lightly season with salt.

4. Add onions to a small bowl, then cover with warm water. Wait 10 minutes, then rinse.

5. In a medium bowl, combine sour cream, mayonnaise, and mustard.

6. Add dressing, onion, celery, pickles, eggs, and herbs to potatoes. Gently stir to combine. Try not to mash the potatoes. Season with salt and pepper.

7. Refrigerate at least 30 minutes before serving. Serve cold or bring to room temperature. You can keep salad refrigerated for up to 3 days.

Serves 6 to 8.

SEAWEED SALAD

Ingredients:
¾ ounce dried organic wakame seaweed
3 tablespoons organic rice vinegar
3 tablespoons organic balsamic vinegar
2 teaspoons organic blackstrap molasses
1 tablespoon organic unrefined sesame oil
1 teaspoon rapadura or granulated maple sugar
Red pepper flakes
1 teaspoon finely grated ginger
½ teaspoon minced garlic
2 scallions, thinly sliced
¼ cup shredded carrot
2 tablespoons chopped fresh cilantro
1 tablespoon sesame seeds, toasted

Directions:
1 Soak seaweed in warm water, enough to cover for 5 minutes. Drain and rinse, then squeeze out excess water. If wakame is uncut, cut into ½-inch-wide strips.

2. Stir together rice vinegar, balsamic vinegar, blackstrap molasses, sesame oil, rapadura or granulated maple sugar, pepper flakes, ginger, and garlic in a bowl. Add the seaweed, scallions, carrots, and cilantro, tossing to combine well. Sprinkle salad with sesame seeds.

Serves 4.

WILD RICE SALAD

Ingredients
1 cup organic wild rice, rinsed
½ cup dried organic cranberries
¾ cup organic pecans, coarsely chopped
2 organic scallions, finely sliced
2 tablespoons organic extra virgin olive oil
2 tablespoons organic apple cider vinegar
¾ teaspoon orange zest and 2 tablespoons juice from one organic orange
1 teaspoon raw organic honey
Celtic or Himalayan sea salt and pepper, to taste

Directions:
1. Add rice, salt, and 3½ cups filtered water to a pot and bring to a boil. Turn heat down to low, cover, and simmer until rice is done, about 50 minutes. Transfer rice to a strainer to drain excess water, then set aside to cool.

2. Combine rice with cranberries, pecans, scallions, olive oil, vinegar, orange zest, orange juice, and honey. Season to taste with salt and pepper, then serve.

Serves 4.

AMARANTH SALAD

Ingredients:
1½ cups cold filtered water
½ cup uncooked whole-grain organic amaranth
2 cups diced unpeeled organic cucumber
½ cup thinly sliced organic celery
½ cup finely chopped organic red onion
¼ cup chopped fresh organic mint
¼ cup chopped fresh flat-leaf organic parsley
¼ cup organic pine nuts, toasted
2 tablespoons organic extra virgin olive oil
1 teaspoon grated organic lemon rind
2 tablespoons fresh organic lemon juice
¼ teaspoon Celtic or Himalayan sea salt
¼ teaspoon crushed red pepper
½ cup drained no-salt-added canned chickpeas
1 cup (4 ounces) organic feta cheese, crumbled

Directions:
1. Bring 1½ cups cold water and amaranth to a boil in a medium saucepan; reduce heat, cover, and simmer for 20 minutes or until the water is almost absorbed.

2. While the amaranth cooks, combine cucumber and the next 11 ingredients in a large bowl.

3. Place amaranth in a fine mesh sieve and rinse under cold running water until room temperature; drain well, pressing with the back of a spoon. Add to cucumber mixture; toss to blend. Add cheese; toss gently.

Serves 4.

MEDITERRANEAN SALAD

Ingredients:
4 cups organic salad greens
2 medium organic tomatoes, chopped
3 medium organic cucumbers, chopped
½ red or purple organic onion, sliced
8 ounces organic feta cheese
Vinaigrette of your choice (or use apple cider vinaigrette)

Directions:
1. Layer salad greens, tomatoes, cucumber, onion, and feta cheese onto a medium serving platter or in a medium bowl.

2. Add a homemade vinaigrette of your choice or apple cider vinaigrette.

Serves 4 to 6.

APPLE CIDER VINAIGRETTE

Ingredients:
1 organic garlic clove, minced
1 tablespoon organic Dijon mustard
¼ cup raw organic apple cider vinegar
2 tablespoons fresh organic lemon juice
2 tablespoons organic raw honey
1/3 cup pure extra virgin olive oil
Celtic or Himalayan sea salt and pepper, to taste

Directions:
1. Combine all the ingredients in a glass mason jar, then seal the lid and shake until the honey dissolves and the ingredients are well combined. For best flavor, allow the dressing to marinate for at least 30 minutes before serving over your salad.

2. Store leftovers in the fridge for up to a week; shake well before serving each time.

Serves 6 to 8.

TUNA SALMON SALAD

Ingredients:

1 large can water-packed tuna fish or 1½ cups cooked wild salmon

3 sticks organic celery, finely chopped

2 organic green onions, finely chopped

4 tablespoons chopped organic parsley or cilantro

½ cup grass-fed cream

2 free-range egg yolks

2 tablespoons wine vinegar

Pinch of Celtic or Himalayan sea salt and freshly ground pepper

Directions:

1. Place the tuna fish or salmon in a bowl and flake it with a fork. Stir in celery, onion, and parsley or cilantro.

2. Mix cream with egg yolks and vinegar. Mix well with the fish mixture and season with unrefined salt and freshly ground pepper.

Serves 2.

FRUIT SALAD

Ingredients:
2/3 cup organic orange juice, freshly squeezed
1/3 cup organic lemon juice, freshly squeezed
1/3 cup rapadura, granulated maple sugar, or coconut palm
sugar
½ teaspoon grated organic orange zest
½ teaspoon grated organic lemon zest
1 teaspoon vanilla extract
2 cups fresh organic pineapple, cubed
2 cups organic strawberries, hulled and sliced
3 organic kiwi fruits, peeled and sliced
2 organic oranges, peeled and sectioned
1 cup organic seedless red grapes
2 cups organic blueberries

Directions:
1. Bring orange juice, lemon juice, sugar, orange zest, and
lemon zest to a boil in a saucepan over medium-high heat.
Reduce heat to medium-low and simmer until slightly thick-
ened, about 5 minutes. Remove from heat and stir in vanilla
extract. Set aside to cool.

2. Place all the fruit in a large, clear glass bowl. Pour the
cooled sauce over the fruit. Cover and refrigerate for 3 to 4
hours before serving.

Serves 8 to 10.

SCRAMBLED EGGS

Ingredients:
1 free-range egg
1 free-range egg yolk
1 tablespoon grass-fed cream
1 tablespoon grass-fed butter
Pinch of dried herbs or 1 teaspoon chopped organic parsley

Directions:
1. Beat egg, egg yolk, and cream with a whisk. Melt butter in a cast iron skillet.

2. Pour in egg mixture and add dried herbs or chopped parsley.

3. Stir with a wooden spoon until eggs have scrambled.

4. Serve with sourdough toast with butter.

Serves 1.

5-GRAIN ENERGY PORRIDGE

Ingredients:
½ cup organic brown rice
½ cup organic quinoa
¼ cup organic amaranth
¼ cup organic millet
¼ cup organic oat bran
¼ cup unsweetened coconut flakes
1 large sweet-tart organic apple (Pink Lady), cut into ¼-inch
pieces
¼ teaspoon ground cinnamon
2 tablespoons organic raw honey
2 tablespoons bee pollen or royal jelly

Directions:
1. Bring brown rice, quinoa, amaranth, millet, oat bran, salt, and 6 cups filtered water to a boil in a medium pot. Reduce heat, partially cover, and simmer, stirring occasionally, until grains are the consistency of porridge (softer and thicker than the usual bowl of oatmeal) and water is fully absorbed, usually about 40 to 50 minutes.

2. Add apple, cinnamon, and honey to skillet and cook, stirring occasionally until apples are browned in spots and tender, about 3 minutes. Serve porridge topped with apples, coconut, bee pollen, and a drizzle of honey.

Serves 4.

AMARANTH

Ingredients:

2 cups amaranth

4 cups filtered water

½ teaspoon Celtic or Himalayan sea salt

2 or 3 tablespoons chopped walnuts or almonds or other nuts

Organic raw honey and organic grass-fed milk to taste

Directions:

1. In a 4-quart heavy saucepan combine the amaranth and the water. Cover the pan and bring the mixture to a boil, whisking occasionally. Using a heatproof rubber spatula, push any seeds clinging to the side of the pot into the liquid, then reduce the heat to low and continue to simmer, covered, until the liquid is fully absorbed, about 20 to 25 minutes. Stir in salt.

2. Remove the pan from the heat and let it stand, covered, 5 to 10 minutes. Top with nuts, honey, and milk.

Serves 4 to 6.

OATMEAL

Ingredients:
2 cups organic old-fashioned rolled oats (not quick oats)
2 cups warm filtered water
2 tablespoons organic apple cider vinegar, lemon juice, or yogurt
1 teaspoon Celtic or Himalayan sea salt

Directions:
1. In a glass container, mix 2 cups oats with 2 cups warm filtered water and 2 tablespoons apple cider vinegar, lemon juice, or yogurt.

2. Cover and leave in a warm place overnight.

3. In the morning bring an additional 2 cups of filtered water to boil. Add the salt and the soaked oatmeal. Bring to a boil and then reduce to a simmer. Cook about 10 minutes, stirring occasionally.

Serves 4.

BROWN RICE

Ingredients:
1 cup organic brown rice
3 cups filtered water
2 tablespoons organic yogurt
4 cups filtered water or chicken broth
4 tablespoons grass-fed butter
1 teaspoon Celtic or Himalayan sea salt

Directions:
1. In the morning, place brown rice in a 1-quart jar with 3 cups water and 2 tablespoons yogurt. Cover tightly and allow to soak in a warm place during the day. Drain the rice through a strainer.

2. Bring 4 cups water or chicken stock to a boil and add the soaked rice, butter, and salt. Bring to a boil and allow to boil uncovered until the level of the water is reduced to the level of the rice.

3. Cover the pan and reduce heat to a simmer. You can cook the rice on the stove top on a burner set to very low or in the oven at 250°. Cook gently for about 2 hours, stirring occasionally.

4. Serve with meat, chicken, or seafood.

Serves 4.

WHOLE-GRAIN PANCAKES

Ingredients:
2 cups organic whole-grain flour
2 cups organic yogurt
2 free-range eggs, beaten
1 teaspoon organic baking soda
2 tablespoons grass-fed butter, melted
¼ cup organic maple syrup

Directions:
1. Mix flour with yogurt; cover and leave in a warm place overnight.

2. In the morning, add remaining ingredients and thin the batter with a little water to desired consistency. Cook in batches on a hot griddle or in a cast-iron pan.

3. Serve with melted butter and maple syrup.

Serves 6 to 8.

BAKED BEANS

Ingredients:
2 cups organic navy beans
1 organic onion, peeled and finely chopped
½ pound organic bacon (optional)
2 pounds organic sausage, sliced
3 tablespoons organic blackstrap molasses
1 small can organic tomato paste
½ teaspoon dry mustard
2 teaspoons Celtic or Himalayan sea salt
¼ teaspoon black pepper
½ cup organic maple syrup

Directions:
1. Soak beans overnight in warm water. Drain the beans and cover again with water. Cook approximately 1 to 2 hours and drain.

2. Arrange the beans in a greased 2-quart pot by placing a portion of the beans in the bottom of the pot and layering them with bacon, onion, and sausage.

3. In a small saucepan, combine remaining ingredients. Bring the mixture to a boil; pour over beans and add additional water to cover the beans.

4. Cover the pot with a lid and bake at 250° for 3 to 4 hours, until beans are tender. Check the pot about halfway through cooking, and add more liquid if necessary to prevent the beans from getting too dry.

Serves 6.

MAPLE SALMON

Ingredients:
¼ cup organic maple syrup
1 tablespoon organic balsamic vinegar
1 tablespoon organic blackstrap molasses
1 clove organic garlic, minced
¼ teaspoon Celtic or Himalayan sea salt
1/8 teaspoon ground black pepper
1 pound wild-caught salmon

Directions:
1. In a small bowl, mix the maple syrup, balsamic vinegar, blackstrap molasses, garlic, salt, and pepper.

2. Place salmon in a shallow glass baking dish and coat with the maple syrup mixture. Cover the dish and marinate salmon in the refrigerator for 30 minutes, turning once.

3. Preheat oven to 400°F (200°C).

4. Place the baking dish in the preheated oven and bake salmon uncovered 20 minutes, or until easily flaked with a fork.

Serves 4.

GRILLED CHICKEN CHILI

Ingredients:
2 skinless organic chicken breasts
1 tablespoon organic extra virgin coconut oil
1½ tablespoon chili sauce
2 teaspoons grated organic ginger
2 tablespoons organic raw honey
2 tablespoons apple cider or rice vinegar
240 grams broccoli
1 tablespoons sesame seeds

Directions:
1. Slice each chicken breast lengthways into 2 thin pieces. Rub with the coconut oil and season on both sides. Heat a grill pan and cook the pieces for 2 to 3 minutes on each side.

2. While the chicken is cooking, mix the chili sauce, ginger, honey, and vinegar with a little seasoning in a small bowl. Brush over the chicken as it cooks—wait until it is grilled on one side first before brushing, or it will burn.

3. Blanch the broccoli, divide between the plates and pour over the remaining sauce. Top with the chicken and sesame seeds.

Serves 2.

GREEK LAMP CHOPS

Ingredients:
1 tablespoon dried oregano
2 tablespoons organic lemon juice
1 tablespoon bottled minced organic garlic
½ teaspoon Celtic or Himalayan sea salt
¼ teaspoon black pepper
8 (4-ounce) organic lamb loin chops, trimmed
Organic extra virgin coconut oil cooking spray

Directions:
1. Preheat broiler.

2. Combine oregano, lemon juice, garlic, sea salt, and black pepper and rub the mixture over both sides of the chops.

3. Place the chops on a broiler pan coated with coconut oil cooking spray; broil 4 minutes on each side or until desired degree of doneness.

Serves 4 (serving size: 2 lamb chops).

KALE CHIPS

Ingredients:

1 bunch of organic kale, washed, dried, and stems removed
1 tablespoon organic extra virgin coconut oil, melted
½ teaspoon garlic powder
¼ teaspoon red chili flakes
⅛ teaspoon ground ginger
Celtic or Himalayan sea salt and pepper to taste

Directions:

1. Preheat oven to 300°F.

2. Cut or tear the kale into smaller pieces so that the chips are not huge. Spread them onto a baking sheet. Pour the melted coconut oil over the kale and massage until all kale leaves are covered. Sprinkle on the garlic, red chili flakes, ginger, salt, and pepper. Toss to combine.

3. Place into the oven and bake for about 15 minutes, then give them a toss. Continue cooking until crispy, 5 to 10 minutes.

Serves 2.

MACAROONS

Ingredients:
4 free-range egg whites
Pinch of Celtic or Himalayan sea salt
½ cup rapadura or granulated maple sugar
1 teaspoon vanilla extract
2 cups unsweetened desiccated coconut (finely cut)

Directions:
1. Line a baking sheet with buttered parchment paper.

2. Beat egg whites with salt in a clean bowl until they form stiff peaks. Gradually work in remaining ingredients.

3. Drop mixture by spoonful onto parchment paper.

4. Bake at 300° for 1/2 hour, then at 200° for 1 hour.

5. Allow to cool before removing from parchment paper.

Makes about 2 dozen.

CHOCOLATE CAKE

Ingredients:
6 free-range eggs
2/3 teaspoon vanilla liquid stevia extract
¼ teaspoon powdered stevia extract
1 cup unsweetened vanilla almond milk
½ cup organic extra virgin coconut oil, melted
½ cup coconut flour
¼ cup almond meal
½ cup unsweetened organic cocoa powder
½ teaspoon Celtic or Himalayan sea salt
¾ teaspoon organic baking soda
2 tablespoons strong organic coffee

Directions:
1. Beat the eggs with the stevia and almond milk until light in color.

2. Beat in the coconut oil and coffee.

3. In a separate bowl, combine the coconut flour, almond meal, cocoa powder, salt, and baking soda.

4. Slowly incorporate the wet ingredients into the dry ingredients, mixing well.

5. Pour the mixture into a 9-inch baking pan lined with parchment paper and bake at 350° for 15 to 20 minutes, or until set in the middle.

Frosting Ingredients:
1/3 cup organic cocoa
2 teaspoons stevia powder
¼ cup organic extra virgin coconut oil, melted
½ cup organic coconut cream, chilled until firm
½ teaspoon vanilla extract

Frosting Instructions:
1. Combine the ingredients in a medium-sized bowl and beat until fluffy.

2. Spread on the cooled cake.

HEALTHIER CHOCOLATE CAKE

Ingredients:
One 15-ounce can (or 15 ounces cooked) unseasoned organic black beans
5 large free-range eggs
1 tablespoon vanilla extract
½ teaspoon Celtic or Himalayan sea salt
6 tablespoons unsalted grass-fed butter
½ cup + 2 tablespoons organic raw honey or another sweetener
6 tablespoons unsweetened organic cocoa powder
2 teaspoons organic baking powder
Organic extra virgin coconut oil cooking spray
Chocolate cake frosting

Directions:
1. Preheat oven to 350°F (163°C).

2. Spray a 9-inch cake pan with coconut oil cooking spray, or grease it with a thin layer of grass-fed butter.

3. Dust cocoa all over the inside of the pan, tapping to evenly distribute.

4. Cut a round of parchment paper and line the bottom of the pan, then grease the parchment lightly. Alternatively, you can make cupcakes. If you'd like to bake the batter as cupcakes, line 16 cupcake tins with paper liners.

5. Drain and rinse beans in a strainer or colander. Shake off excess water.

6. Place beans, 3 of the eggs, vanilla, and salt into a blender.

7. Blend on high until beans are completely liquefied. Whisk together cocoa powder and baking powder.

8. In a bowl, use a mixer to cream the butter with sweetener (erythritol or honey) until light and fluffy.

9. Mix in the 2 remaining eggs, beating for a minute after each addition.

10. Beat the bean mixture into the rest of the batter.

11. Stir in cocoa powder and water, and beat the batter on high for one minute, until smooth.

12. Scrape batter into pan and smooth the top.

13. Grip pan firmly by the edges and rap it on the counter a few times to pop any air bubbles.

14. If you are baking the cake as a single round layer, bake for 40 to 45 minutes. If you are baking the batter as cupcakes, bake for 35 minutes. The cake is done when the top springs back when you press on it.

15. Remove cake to a cooling rack to cool for 10 minutes.

16. Turn out the cake from pan and flip over again onto cooling rack.

17. Let cake cool until it reaches room temperature, then cover with plastic wrap. For best flavor, let the cake sit overnight.

18. If you are stacking this cake, level the top with a long serrated knife, shaving off layers until the cake round is flat and even.

19. Store cake or cupcakes in the refrigerator. For the best flavor and texture, warm the cake to room temperature before serving.

Frosting Ingredients:
½ cup (1 stick) unsalted grass-fed butter, softened
¼ cup powdered erythritol and 1 tablespoon powdered xylitol
6 tablespoons unsweetened organic cocoa powder
2 tablespoons grass-fed half and half or coconut milk
1 teaspoon vanilla extract
1 free-range egg yolk
Pinch of Celtic or Himalayan sea salt
Pure stevia extract, to taste

Frosting Directions:
1. Cream the butter in a small bowl until fluffy.

2. Powder erythritol and xylitol in a coffee grinder or Magic Bullet for a minute or two, until extremely fine in texture (reminiscent of powdered sugar).

3. Stir powdered sweetener into butter with a spatula, then beat until smooth.

4. Slowly blend in the cocoa powder, vanilla, and sea salt.

5. Beat in the egg yolk and grass-fed half and half or coconut milk.

6. Add stevia, starting with 1/16 teaspoon. Keep tasting and adjusting the sweetness to your liking.

CHOCOLATE CHIP COOKIES

Ingredients:
2 cups organic whole-grain flour or flour substitute
¾ teaspoon Celtic or Himalayan sea salt
¾ teaspoon organic baking powder
1 free-range egg
½ teaspoon stevia powder
1 teaspoon vanilla extract
1 cup salted grass-fed butter, softened
1¼ cups organic chocolate chips

Directions:
1. Preheat oven to 350°F (180°C).

2. Lightly grease a cookie sheet and set aside. In a medium mixing bowl, sift together the flour, salt, and baking powder, and set aside.

3 Place the egg, stevia, and vanilla in a large mixing bowl. Beat well with a wooden spoon or electric hand-held mixer.

4. Slowly add the butter, continuing to beat until the mixture is smooth and creamy.

5. Add the flour mixture to the butter mixture, ½ cup at a time, stirring well with a wooden spoon after each addition. Fold in the chocolate chips.

6. Drop heaping teaspoons of batter on the cookie sheet, about 2 inches apart.

7. Bake for 20 to 25 minutes, or until the cookies are golden brown.

Yields 50 cookies.

ALMOND FLOUR CAKE

Ingredients:
2 sticks grass-fed butter, softened
2 tablespoons stevia powder
15 drops stevia liquid
5 free-range eggs, room temperature
2 cups organic almond flour
1 teaspoon organic baking powder
1 teaspoon lemon extract
1 teaspoon vanilla extract

Directions:
1. Cream butter and stevia well. Add eggs one at a time, beating well after each.

2 Mix almond flour with baking powder, then add a little at a time to the egg mixture, beating as you do so. Add lemon and vanilla extracts.

3. Pour mixture into a greased 9-inch square pan. Bake at 350°F for 45 to 50 minutes.

Note: For a creamier cake, use 1 stick of butter and ½ cup of softened, full-fat grass-fed cream cheese.

ALMOND COOKIES

Ingredients:

1 cup almond meal or almond flour
¼ cup unsweetened shredded organic coconut
2 teaspoons almond extract
¼ cup organic extra virgin coconut oil
2 tablespoons raw almond butter
¼ teaspoon Celtic or Himalayan sea salt
30 drops clear liquid stevia extract

Directions:

1. Preheat oven to 325°F (160°C).

2. Combine all ingredients in a medium bowl and stir until you have a soft ball of dough. Scoop by the tablespoon-full onto a parchment-lined cookie sheet.

3. Bake for 60 to 90 minutes until golden.

5. Remove from oven and cool completely. Store in refrigerator.

COCONUT MILK ICE CREAM

Ingredients:
1 can full-fat organic coconut milk (13.5 ounces)
3 frozen organic bananas or ½ cup coconut palm sugar
A pinch of sea salt

Directions:
1. Blend coconut milk with your sugar of choice (frozen bananas or coconut palm sugar) and extract flavorings in a high-speed blender.

2. Pour into a (pre-frozen) ice cream machine. Mix for at least 20 minutes.

3. Stir in chopped nuts, cacao nibs, or cookies, depending on which flavor you want. Best served immediately; if stored in the freezer, place back in the ice cream maker to make it smooth and creamy again.

Almond Pistachio Flavor: 1½ teaspoon almond extract, 1 vanilla bean seeded or 1 teaspoon vanilla extract, ½ cup toasted and chopped almonds and pistachios

Mint Chocolate Chip Flavor: 2 teaspoons peppermint extract, ⅓ cup raw organic cacao nibs or chocolate chips of your choice

Cookies and Cream Flavor: 1 tablespoon vanilla extract, 10 cacao cookies broken into pieces or a cookie of your choice

Serves 10.

BETTER THAN COFFEE

Ingredients:

1 tablespoon Cafix, Dandy Blend, or another coffee substitute

1 tablespoon grass-fed cream

1 teaspoon organic maple syrup or organic raw honey (optional)

Directions:

1. Place 1 tablespoon coffee substitute in a mug and pour in boiling water.

2. Stir in the cream. Let cool slightly and add sweetener.

Serves 1.

REFERENCES

PREFACE

1. Rodin, J., Radke-Sharpe, N., Rebuffé-Scrive, M., & Greenwood, M. R. (1990). Weight cycling and fat distribution. *International Journal of Obesity,* 14(4), 303–10.

2. Van der Kooy, K., Leenen, R., Seidell, J. C., Deurenberg, P., & Hautvast, J. G. (1993). Effect of a weight cycle on visceral fat accumulation. *American Journal of Clinical Nutrition,* 58(6), 853–57.

3. World Health Organization Technical Report Series. (2003). *Diet, nutrition and the prevention of chronic diseases.* 916, 1-149.

INTRODUCTION

1. NIH Technology Assessment Conference Panel. (1993). *Methods for voluntary weight loss and control. Ann Int Med,* 119, 688-693.

2. Lustig A. (1991). Weight loss programs: failing to meet ethical standards? *J Am Dietetic Assoc,* 91, 1252-1254.

3. Strychar, I. (2006). Diet in the management of weight loss. *CMAJ,* 174 (1), 56–63.

4. Bacon, L., & Aphramor, L. (2011). Weight science: evaluating the evidence for a paradigm shift. *Nutr J,* 10, 9.

5. Andreasen, C. H., Stender-Petersen, K. L., Mogensen, & M. S. (2008). Low physical activity accentuates the effect of the FTO rs9939609 polymorphism on body fat accumulation. *Diabetes,* 57, 95-101.

6. Kilpeläinen, T. O., Qi, L., & Brage, S. (2011). Physical activity attenuates the influence of FTO variants on obesity

risk: a meta-analysis of 218,166 adults and 19,268 children. *PLoS Med,* 8(11), e1001116.

7. Popkin, B.M., & Duffey, K.J. (2010). Does hunger and satiety drive eating anymore? Increasing eating occasions and decreasing time between eating occasions in the United States. *Am J Clin Nutr,* 91, 1342-7.

8. David, M. Cutler, Edward, L., Glaeser, Jesse, M., & Shapiro. (2003). Why Have Americans Become More Obese? NBER Working Papers 9446. *National Bureau of Economic Research, Inc.*

9. David, M., Cutler, Edward, L., Glaeser, Jesse, M., & Shapiro. (2003). Why Have Americans Become More Obese? NBER Working Papers 9446. *National Bureau of Economic Research, Inc.*

10. Swanson, D.W., & Dinello, F.A. (1970). Follow-up of patients starved for obesity. *Psychosom Med,* 32(2), 209-14.

11. Stice, E., Burger, K., & Yokum, S. (2013). Caloric deprivation increases responsivity of attention and reward brain regions to intake, anticipated intake, and images of palatable foods. *Neuroimage,* 67, 322-30.

12. Tomiyama, A. J, Mann, T., & Vinas, D. (2010). Low calorie dieting increases cortisol. *Psychosom Med,* 72(4), 357-64.

13. Kohsaka, A., Laposky, A.D., & Ramsey, K.M. (2007). High-fat diet disrupts behavioral and molecular circadian rhythms in mice. *Cell Metab,* 6(5), 414-21.

14. Arble, D.M., Bass, J., Laposky, A.D., Vitaterna, M.H., & Turek FW. (2009). Circadian timing of food intake contributes to weight gain. *Obesity,* 17, 2100–2102.

15. Goel, N., Stunkard, A.J., & Rogers, N.L. (2009). Circadian rhythm profiles in women with night eating syndrome. *J Biol Rhythms,* 24, 85–94.

16. Buxton, O.M., Cain, S.W., & O'Connor, S.P. (2012). Adverse metabolic consequences in humans of prolonged sleep restriction combined with circadian disruption. *Sci Transl Med,* 4(129), 129ra43.

17. Ellenbroek, J.H., Van Dijck, L., & Töns, H.A. (2014). Long-term ketogenic diet causes glucose intolerance and reduced β- and α-cell mass but no weight loss in mice. *Am J Physiol Endocrinol Metab,* 306(5), E552-8.

18. Brownell, K.D., & Rodin, J. (1994). Medical, metabolic, and psychological effects of weight cycling. *Arch Intern Med,* 154(12). 1325-30.

19. Rzehak, P., Meisinger, C., & Woelke G. (2007). Weight change, weight cycling and mortality in the ERFORT Male Cohort Study. *Eur J Epidemiol,* 22(10), 665-73.

20. Kiefer, A., Lin, J., Blackburn, E., & Epel, E. (2008). Dietary restraint and telomere length in pre- and postmenopausal women. *Psychosom Med,* 70(8), 845-9.

21. Tomiyama, A.J., O'Donovan, A., Lin, J., & Puterman, E. (2012). Does cellular aging relate to patterns of allostasis? An examination of basal and stress reactive HPA axis activity and telomere length. *Physiol Behav,* 106(1), 40-5.

22. Taylor, E., Missik, E., Hurley, R., Hudak, S., & Logue, E. (2004). Obesity treatment: broadening our perspective. *Am J Health Behav,* 28, 242–249.

23. Jakubowicz, D., Froy, O., Wainstein, J., Boaz, M. (2012). Meal timing and composition influence ghrelin levels, appetite scores and weight loss maintenance in overweight and obese adults. *Steroids,* 77(4), 323-31.

24. Garaulet, M., Gómez-Abellán, P. (2014). Timing of food intake and obesity: a novel association. *Physiol Behav,* 134, 44-50.

25. Mattson, M. P. (2014). Meal frequency and timing in health and disease. *Proc Natl Acad Sci U S A,* 111(47), 16647-53.

26. Bandín, C., Martinez-Nicolas, A., Ordovás, J.M., Madrid, J.A., & Garaulet, M. (2014). Circadian rhythmicity as a predictor of weight-loss effectiveness. *Int J Obes (Lond),* 38(8), 1083-8.

CHAPTER 1: EATING HABITS

1. Tai, M.M., Castillo, P., & Pi-Sunyer, F.X. (1991). Meal size and frequency: effect on the thermic effect of food. *Am J Clin Nutr,* 54, 783–787.

2. Kahleova, H., Belinova, L., & Malinska, H. (2014). Eating two larger meals a day (breakfast and lunch) is more effective than six smaller meals in a reduced-energy regimen for patients with type 2 diabetes: a randomised crossover study. *Diabetologia,* 57(8), 1552–1560.

3. Schoenfeld, B.J., Aragon, A.A., & Krieger, J.W. (2015). Effects of meal frequency on weight loss and body composition: a meta-analysis. *Nutrition Reviews,* 73, 69-82.

4. Kant, A. K. (2014). Evidence for efficacy and effectiveness of changes in eating frequency for body weight management. *Adv Nutr,* 5(6), 822-8.

5. Duffey, K. J., & Popkin, B. M. (2011). Energy density, portion size, and eating occasions: contributions to increased energy intake in the United States, 1977-2006. *PLoS Med,* 8(6), e1001050.

6. Bellisle, F., McDevitt, R., & Prentice, A. M. (1997). Meal frequency and energy balance. *Br J Nutr,* 77 Suppl 1, S57-70.

7. Howarth, N. C., Huang, T., & Roberts, S. B. (2007). Eating patterns and dietary composition in relation to BMI in younger and older adults. *Int J Obes,* 31(4), 675-84.

8. Mattson, M.P. (2005). Energy intake, meal frequency, and health: a neurobiological perspective. *Annu Rev Nutr,* 25, 237-60.

9. Richards, B. (2009). *Mastering Leptin: Your Guide to Permanent Weight Loss and Optimum Health.* Wellness Resources.

10. Cowan, T. (2004). *The Fourfold Path to Healing: Working with the Laws of Nutrition, Therapeutics, Movement and Meditation in the Art of Medicine.* Newtrends Publishing.

11. Innes, E. (2014, March 31). *The best times to eat breakfast, lunch and dinner if you want to lose weight - and you need to make sure you're up by 7am.* Retrieved from http://www.dailymail.co.uk/health/article-2593219/Revealed-The-best-times-eat-breakfast-lunch-dinner-want-lose-weight-need-make-sure-youre-7am.html#ixzz3erswq8Zm

12. Garaulet, M., & Gómez-Abellán, P. (2014). Timing of food intake and obesity: a novel association. *Physiol Behav,* 134, 44-50.

13. Garaulet, M., Gómez-Abellán, P., & Alburquerque-Béjar, J.J. (2013). Timing of food intake predicts weight loss effectiveness. *Int J Obes (Lond),* 37, 604–611.

14. Bandín, C., Scheer, F.A., & Luque, A.J. (2015). Meal timing affects glucose tolerance, substrate oxidation and circadian-related variables: A randomized, crossover trial. *Int J Obes (Lond),* 39(5), 828-33.

15. Davis, C., Curtis, C., Tweed, S., & Patte, K. (2007). Psychological factors associated with ratings of portion size: relevance to the risk profile for obesity. *Eat Behav,* 8(2), 170–176.

16. Heymsfield, S.B., Van Mierlo, C. A., Van der Knaap, H. C., Heo, M., & Frier, H. I. (2003). Weight management using a meal replacement strategy: meta and pooling analysis from six studies. *Int J Obes Relat Metab Disord,* 27(5), 537-549.

17. Tsai, A. G., & Wadden, T. A. (2006). The evolution of very-low-calorie diets: an update and meta-analysis. *Obesity,* 14(8), 1283-1293.

18. Ruge, T., Hodson, L., & Cheeseman, J. (2009). Fasted to fed trafficking of fatty acids in human adipose tissue reveals a novel regulatory step for enhanced fat storage. *J Clin Endocrinol Metab,* 94, 1781–1788.

19. Wheeler, K. (2014). *The Marie Antoinette Diet: How to Eat Cake and Still Lose Weight.* Sweet Pea Publishing.

20. Pedersen, C.R., Hagemann, I., Bock, T., & Buschard, K. (1999). Intermittent feeding and fasting reduces diabetes incidence in BB rats. *Autoimmunity,* 30, 243–250.

21. Fernemark, H., Jaredsson, C., & Bunjaku, B. (2013, November 27). A randomized cross-over trial of the postprandial effects of three different diets in patients with type 2 diabetes. *PLoS One,* 8(11), e79324.

22. Douillard, J., (2011, December 22). *Dangers of Frequent Eating.* Retrieved from http://lifespa.com/dangers-of-frequent-eating/

23. Johnstone, A. (2015). Fasting for weight loss: an effective strategy or latest dieting trend? *Int J Obes (Lond),* 39(5), 727-733.

24. Johnstone, A.M. (2007). Fasting - the ultimate diet? *Obes Rev,* 8(3), 211-22.

25. Harvie, M., Wright, C., & Pegington, M. (2013). The effect of intermittent energy and carbohydrate restriction v. daily energy restriction on weight loss and metabolic disease risk markers in overweight women. *Br J Nutr,* 110(8), 1534-47.

26. Kim, I., Lemasters, J.J. (2011). Mitochondrial degradation by autophagy (mitophagy) in GFP-LC3 transgenic hepatocytes during nutrient deprivation. *Am J Physiol Cell Physiol,* 300(2), C308-17.

27. Cuervo, E., Bergamini, U.T., Brunk, W., Droge, M., French, A., & Terman. (2005). Autophagy and aging: the importance of maintaining "clean" cells. *Autophagy,* 1(3), 131-40.

28. Glynn, E.L., Fry, C.S., Drummond, M.J., Timmerman, K.L., Dhanani, S., Volpi, E., & Rasmussen, B.B. (2010). Excess leucine intake enhances muscle anabolic signaling but not net protein anabolism in young men and women. *J Nutr,* 140(11), 1970-6.

29. Jaeger, P.A., & Wyss-Coray, T. (2009). All-you-can-eat: autophagy in neurodegeneration and neuroprotection. *Mol Neurodegener,* 4, 16.

30. Ding, W.X. (2011). The emerging role of autophagy in alcoholic liver disease. *Exp Biol Med,* 546-556.

31. Aly, S.M. (2014). Role of intermittent fasting on improving health and reducing diseases. *Int J Health Sci (Qassim),* 8(3), V-VI.

32. Anton, S., & Leeuwenburgh, C. (2013). Fasting or caloric restriction for healthy aging. *Exp Gerontol,* 48(10), 1003-5.

33. Wegman, M.P., Guo, M.H., & Bennion, D.M. (2015). Practicality of intermittent fasting in humans and its effect on oxidative stress and genes related to aging and metabolism. *Rejuvenation Res,* 18(2), 162-72.

34. Skaznik-Wikiel, M.E., & Polotsky, A.J. (2014).The health pros and cons of continuous versus intermittent calorie restriction: more questions than answers. *Maturitas,* 79(3), 275-8.

35. Longo, V.D., & Mattson, M.P. (2014). Fasting: molecular mechanisms and clinical applications. *Cell Metab,* 19(2), 181-92.

36. Barnosky, A.R., Hoddy, K.K., Unterman, T.G., & Varady KA. (2014). Intermittent fasting vs daily calorie restriction for type 2 diabetes prevention: a review of human findings. *Transl Res,* 164(4), 302-11.

37. Mattson, M.P., & Wan, R. (2005). Beneficial effects of intermittent fasting and caloric restriction on the cardiovascular and cerebrovascular systems. *J Nutr Biochem,* 16, 129–37.

38. Mattison, J.A., Lane, M.A., Roth, G.S., & Ingram, D.K. (2003). Calorie restriction in rhesus monkeys. *Exp Gerontol,* 38, 35–46.

39. Ahmet, I., Wan, R., Mattson, M.P., Lakatta, E.G., & Talan, M. (2005). Cardioprotection by intermittent fasting in rats. *Circulation,* 112, 3115–21.

40. Anson, R.M., Guo, Z., & de Cabo, R. (2003). Intermittent fasting dissociates beneficial effects of dietary restriction on glucose metabolism and neuronal resistance to injury from calorie intake. *Proc Natl Acad Sci U S A,* 100, 6216–20.

41. Berrigan, D., Perkins, S.N., Haines, D.C., & Hursting, S.D. (2002). Adult-onset calorie restriction and fasting delay

spontaneous tumorigenesis in p53-deficient mice. *Carcinogenesis,* 23, 817–22.

42. Sohal, R.S., & Weindruch, R. (1996). Oxidative stress, caloric restriction, and aging. *Science,* 273, 59–63.

43. Speakman, J.R., Selman, C., McLaren, J.S., & Harper, E.J. (2002). Living fast, dying when? The link between aging and energetics. *J Nutr,* 132 (suppl), 1583S–97S.

44. Roth, G.S., Ingram, D.K., & Lane, M.A. (2001). Caloric restriction in primates and relevance to humans. *Ann N Y Acad Sci,* 928, 305–15.

45. Sebastian, B., In, Y. C., Min, W., & Chia, W.C. (2015). A Periodic Diet that Mimics Fasting Promotes Multi-System Regeneration, Enhanced Cognitive Performance, and Healthspan. *Cell Metabolism,* 22(1), 86–99.

46. Brown, J.E. (2014). Can restricting calories help you to live longer? *Post Reprod Health,* 20(1), 16-18.

47. Michalsen, A., & Li, C. (2013). Fasting therapy for treating and preventing disease - current state of evidence. *Forsch Komplementmed,* 20(6), 444-53.

48. Trepanowski, J.F., & Bloomer, R.J. (2010). The impact of religious fasting on human health. *Nutr J,* 9, 57.

49. Berg, J. M., Tymoczko, J. L., & Stryer, L. (2002). Food Intake and Starvation Induce Metabolic Changes. In *Biochemistry (5th edition).* New York: W H Freeman.

50. Moritz, A. (2005). *Timeless Secrets of Health and Rejuvenation.* Ener-chi.

51. Koopmann. (2014). Hypercaloric diets with increased meal frequency, but not meal size, increase intrahepatic tri-

glycerides: A randomized controlled trial. *Hepatology*, 60(2), 545-53.

52. Rothschild, A., Hoddy, K. K., Jambazian, P., Varady, K. A. (2014). Time Restricted Feeding and Risk of Metabolic Disease: A Review of Human and Animal Studies. *Nutrition Reviews*, 72(5), 308-318.

53. Mattson, M.P. (2005). ENERGY intake, meal frequency, and health: a neurobiological perspective. *Annu Rev Nutr*, 25, 237–260.

54. Anson, R.M., Guo, Z., & de Cabo, R. (2003). Intermittent fasting dissociates beneficial effects of dietary restriction on glucose metabolism and neuronal resistance to injury from calorie intake. *Proc Natl Acad Sci U S A*, 100, 6216–6220.

55. Hatori, M., Vollmers, C., & Zarrinpar, A. (2012). Time-restricted feeding without reducing caloric intake prevents metabolic diseases in mice fed a high-fat diet. *Cell Metab*, 15, 848–860.

56. Sherman, H., Genzer, Y., & Cohen, R. (2012). Timed high-fat diet resets circadian metabolism and prevents obesity. *FASEB J*, 26, 3493–3502.

57. Chaix, A., Zarrinpar, A., Miu, P., & Panda, S. (2014). Time-Restricted Feeding Is a Preventative and Therapeutic Intervention against Diverse Nutritional Challenges. *Cell Metabolism*, 20(6), 991-1005.

58. Cheng, K., Andrikopoulos, S., & Gunton, J.E. (2013). First phase insulin secretion and type 2 diabetes. *Curr Mol Med*, 13(1), 126-39.

59. Farshchi, H. R., Taylor, M. A., Macdonald, I. A. (2004). Regular meal frequency creates more appropriate insulin sensitivity and lipid profiles compared with irregular meal

frequency in healthy lean women. *Eur J Clin Nutr*, 58(7), 1071-7.

60. Farshchi, H. R., Taylor, M. A., Macdonald, I. A. (2004). Decreased thermic effect of food after an irregular compared with a regular meal pattern in healthy lean women. *Int J Obes Relat Metab Disord*, 28, 653–660.

61. Kahleova, H., Belinova, L., & Malinska, H. (2014). Eating two larger meals a day (breakfast and lunch) is more effective than six smaller meals in a reduced-energy regimen for patients with type 2 diabetes: a randomised crossover study. *Diabetologia*, 57(8), 1552-60.

62. Lane, J.D., Barkauskas, C.E., Surwit, R.S., & Feinglos, M.N. (2004). Caffeine impairs glucose metabolism in type 2 diabetes. *Diabetes Care*, 27(8), 2047-8.

63. Van Dam, R.M., Pasman, W.J., & Verhoef, P. (2004). Effects of coffee consumption on fasting blood glucose and insulin concentrations: randomized controlled trials in healthy volunteers. *Diabetes Care*, 27(12), 2990-2.

64. Lane, J.D. (2011). Caffeine, Glucose Metabolism, and Type 2 Diabetes. *Journal of Caffeine Research*, 1(1), 23-28.

65. Rodin, J. (1985). Insulin levels, hunger, and food intake: an example of feedback loops in body weight regulation. *Health Psychol*, 4(1), 1-24.

66. Mann, T. (2015). *Secrets from the Eating Lab: The Science of Weight Loss, the Myth of Willpower, and Why You Should Never Diet Again*. New York: HarperWave.

67. Brand-Miller, J.C., Holt, S.H., Pawlak, D.B., & McMillan, J. (2002). Glycemic index and obesity. *Am J Clin Nutr*, 76(1), 281S-5S.

68. Mansell, P.I., Fellows, I.W., & Macdonald, I.A. (1990). Enhanced thermogenic response to epinephrine after 48-h starvation in humans. *Am J Physiol,* 258(1 Pt 2), R87-93.

69. Zauner, C., Schneeweiss, B., & Kranz, A. (2000). Resting energy expenditure in short-term starvation is increased as a result of an increase in serum norepinephrine. *Am J Clin Nutr,* 71(6), 1511-5.

70. Stote, K.S., Baer, D.J., & Spears, K. (2007). A controlled trial of reduced meal frequency without caloric restriction in healthy, normal-weight, middle-aged adults. *Am J Clin Nutr,* 85(4), 981-8.

71. Elfhag, K., Rossner, S. (2005). Who succeeds in maintaining weight loss? A conceptual review of factors associated with weight loss maintenance and weight regain. *Obes Rev,* 6, 67–85.

72. Colles, S.L., Dixon, J.B., & O'Brien, P.E. (2007). Night eating syndrome and nocturnal snacking: association with obesity, binge eating and psychological distress. *Int J Obes (Lond),* 31, 1722–1730.

73. O'Reardon, J. P., Ringel, B. L., & Dinges, D. F. (2004). Circadian eating and sleeping patterns in the night eating syndrome. *Obes Res,* 12(11), 1789–1796.

74. Ma, Y., Bertone, E. R., & Stanek, E. J. (2003). Association between eating patterns and obesity in a free-living US adult population. *Am J Epidemiol,* 158(1), 85–92.

75. Wang, S., Yang, L., Lu, J., Mu, Y. (2015). High-protein breakfast promotes weight loss by suppressing subsequent food intake and regulating appetite hormones in obese Chinese adolescents. *Horm Res Paediatr,* 83(1), 19-25. Farshchi, H. R., Taylor, M. A., & Macdonald, I. A. (2005). Deleterious effects of omitting breakfast on insulin sensitivity and fasting

lipid profiles in healthy lean women. *Am J Clin Nutr,* 81(2), 388-96.

76. Smith, K. J., Gall, S. L., & McNaughton, S. A. (2010). Skipping breakfast: longitudinal associations with cardiometabolic risk factors in the Childhood Determinants of Adult Health Study. *Am J Clin Nutr,* 92(6), 1316-25.

77. Arble, D. M., Bass, J., Laposky, A. D., Vitaterna, M. H., Turek, F. W. (2009). Circadian timing of food intake contributes to weight gain. *Obesity,* 17(11), 2100-2.

78. Summa, K. C., Turek, F. W. (2014). Chronobiology and obesity: Interactions between circadian rhythms and energy regulation. *Adv Nutr,* 5(3), 312S-9S.

79. Laposky, A. D., Bass, J., Kohsaka, A., Turek, F. W. (2008). Sleep and circadian rhythms: key components in the regulation of energy metabolism. *FEBS Lett,* 582(1), 142-51.

80. Turek. (2005). Obesity and metabolic syndrome in circadian Clock mutant mice. *Science,* 308(5724), 1043-5.

81. Jakubowicz, D., Barnea, M., Wainstein, J., Froy, O. (2013). High caloric intake at breakfast vs. dinner differentially influences weight loss of overweight and obese women. *Obesity,* 21(12), 2504-12.

82. Purslow, L. R., Sandhu, M. S., Forouhi, N., et al. (2008). Energy intake at breakfast and weight change: prospective study of 6,764 middle-aged men and women. *Am J Epidemiol,* 167(2), 188-192.

83. Pereira, M. A., Erickson, E., & McKee, P. (2011). Breakfast frequency and quality may affect glycemia and appetite in adults and children. *J Nutr,* 141(1), 163-8.

84. Cahill, L. E., Chiuve, S. E., & Mekary, R. A. (2013). Prospective study of breakfast eating and incident coronary

heart disease in a cohort of male US health professionals. *Circulation*, 128(4), 337-43.

85. Adolphus, K., Lawton, C. L., & Dye, L. (2013). The effects of breakfast on behavior and academic performance in children and adolescents. *Front Hum Neurosci, 7*, 425.

86. Rabinovitz, H. R., Boaz, M., & Ganz, T. (2014). Big breakfast rich in protein and fat improves glycemic control in type 2 diabetics. *Obesity, 22*(5), E46-54.

87. Kamada, I., Truman, L., Bold, J., & Mortimore, D. (2011). The impact of breakfast in metabolic and digestive health. *Gastroenterol Hepatol Bed Bench, 4*(2), 76-85.

88. Kamada, I., Truman, L., Bold, J., & Mortimore, D. (2011). The impact of breakfast in metabolic and digestive health. *Gastroenterol Hepatol Bed Bench, 4*(2), 76–85.

89. Berkey, C.S., Rockett, H.R., Willett, W.C., & Colditz, G.A. (2005). Milk, dairy fat, dietary calcium, and weight gain: a longitudinal study of adolescents. *Arch Pediatr Adolesc Med, 159*(6), 543-50.

90. Jakubowicz, D., Froy, O., Wainstein, J., & Boaz, M. (2012). Meal timing and composition influence ghrelin levels, appetite scores and weight loss maintenance in overweight and obese adults. *Steroids, 77*(4), 323-31.

91. Blom, W. A., Lluch, A., Stafleu, A., Vinoy, S., Holst, J. J., Schaafsma, G., & Hendriks, H. F. (2006). Effect of a high-protein breakfast on the postprandial ghrelin response. *Am J Clin Nutr, 83*(2), 211-20.

92. Bell, E.A., Castellanos, V.H., Pelkman, C.L., Thorwart, M.L., & Rolls BJ. (1998). Energy density of foods affects energy intake in normal-weight women. *American Journal of Clinical Nutrition, 67*, 412-420.

93. Rolls, B.J., Bell, E.A., Castellanos, V.H., Chow, M., Pelkman, C.L., & Thorwart, M.L. (1999). Energy density but not fat content of foods affected energy intake in lean and obese women. *American Journal of Clinical Nutrition,* 69, 863-871.

94. Duncan, K.H., Bacon, J.A., & Weinsier, R.L. (1983). The effects of high and low energy density diets on satiety, energy intake, and eating time of obese and nonobese subjects. *Am J Clin Nutr,* 37(5), 763-7.

95. Ello-Martin, J.A., Roe, L.S., & Rolls, B.J. (2004). A diet reduced in energy density results in greater weight loss than a diet reduced in fat. *Obes Res,* 12, A23

96. Ello-Martin, J.A., Roe, L.S., Ledikwe, J.H., Beach, A.M., & Rolls, B.J. (2007). Dietary energy density in the treatment of obesity: a year-long trial comparing 2 weight-loss diets. *Am J Clin Nutr,* 85(6), 1465-77.

97. Fitzwater, S.L., Weinsier, R.L., Wooldridge, N.H., Birch, R., Liu, C., & Bartolucci, A.A. (1991). Evaluation of long-term weight changes after a multidisciplinary weight control program. *Journal of the American Dietetic Association,* 91, 421-426, 429.

98. Stamler, J., & Dolecek, T.A. (1997). Relation of food and nutrient intakes to body mass in the special intervention and usual care groups in the Multiple Risk Factor Intervention Trial. *American Journal of Clinical Nutrition,* 65, 366S-373S.

99. Ello-Martin, J.A., Roe, L.S., & Rolls, B.J. (2004). A diet reduced in energy density results in greater weight loss than a diet reduced in fat. *Obesity Research,* 12, A23.

100. Spill, M.K., Birch, L.L., Roe, L.S., & Rolls, B.J. (2011). Serving large portions of vegetable soup at the start of a meal

affected children's energy and vegetable intake. *Appetite,* 57(1), 213-9.

101. Rolls, B.J., Fedoroff, I.C., Guthrie, J.F., & Laster, L.J. (1990). Foods with different satiating effects in humans. *Appetite,* 15(2), 115-26.

102. Flood, J.E., & Rolls, B.J. (2007). Soup preloads in a variety of forms reduce meal energy intake. *Appetite,* 49(3), 626-34.

103. Flood-Obbagy, J.E., & Rolls, B.J. (2009). The effect of fruit in different forms on energy intake and satiety at a meal. *Appetite,* 52(2), 416-22.

104. Roe, L.S., Meengs, J.S., & Rolls, B.J. (2012). Salad and satiety. The effect of timing of salad consumption on meal energy intake. *Appetite,* 58(1), 242-8.

105. Xiang, Y.Q. (2008). Mogrosides extract from Siraitia grosvenori scavenges free radicals in vitro and lowers oxidative stress, serum glucose, and lipid levels in alloxan-induced diabetic mice. *Nutrition Research,* 28(4) 278-284.

106. FAQs: *Questions about Xylitol.* Retrived from http://xylitol.org/faqs-questions-about-xylitol

107. Nazir, L., Samad, F., Haroon, W., Kidwai, S., Siddiqi, S., & Zehravi, M. (2014). Comparison of glycaemic response to honey and glucose in type 2 diabetes. *J Pak Med Assoc,* 64(1), 69-71.

CHAPTER 2: DIET
1. Thomas, D. E., Elliott, E. J., & Baur, L. (2007). Low glycaemic index or low glycaemic load diets for overweight and obesity. *Cochrane Database Syst Rev,* 18, (3), CD005105.

2. Brand-Miller, J., McMillan-Price, J., Steinbeck, K., & Caterson, I. (2008). Carbohydrates--the good, the bad and the whole grain. *Asia Pac J Clin Nutr*, 17 Suppl 1, 16-9.

3. Weston A. P. (2009). *Nutrition and Physical Degeneration*. Price Pottenger Nutrition.

4. Fallon, S. (1999). *Nourishing Traditions: The Cookbook that Challenges Politically Correct Nutrition and the Diet Dictocrats*. NewTrends Publishing, Inc.

5. Esposito, K., Kastorini, C. M., Panagiotakos, D. B., & Giugliano, D. (2011). Mediterranean diet and weight loss: meta-analysis of randomized controlled trials. *Metabolic Syndrome and Related Disorders*, 9(1), 1-12.

6. Beunza, J. J. (2010). Adherence to the Mediterranean diet, long-term weight change, and incident overweight or obesity: the Seguimiento Universidad de Navarra (SUN) cohort. *American Journal of Clinical Nutrition*, 92(6), 1484-2493.

7. Romaguera, D. (2010). Mediterranean dietary patterns and prospective weight change in participants of the EPIC-PANACEA project. *American Journal of Clinical Nutrition*, 92(4), 912–21.

8. Shai I. (2008). Weight loss with a low-carbohydrate, Mediterranean, or low-fat diet. *New England Journal of Medicine*, 359(3), 229–41.

9. Knoops, K. T. (2004). Mediterranean diet, lifestyle factors, and 10-year mortality in elderly European men and women: The HALE project. *Journal of the American Medical Association*, 292(12), 1433–39.

10. von Schacky, C. (2002, January 24). Omega-3-fatty acids, Mediterranean cooking, low-fat diet. What really prevents myocardial infarct? *MMW Fortschr Med*, 144(3-4), 37-9.

11. Rosenthal., & Robert, L. (2000). Effectiveness of altering serum cholesterol levels without drugs. *Proc (Bayl Univ Med Cent)*, 13(4), 351-355.

12. Pawlak, D.B., Kushner, J.A., & Ludwig, D.S. (2004). Effects of dietary glycaemic index on adiposity, glucose homoeostasis, and plasma lipids in animals. *Lancet*, 364 (9436), 778-85.

13. Thomas, D.E., Elliott, E.J., & Baur, L. (2007, July 18). Low glycaemic index or low glycaemic load diets for overweight and obesity. *Cochrane Database Syst Rev*, (3), CD005105.

14. Chiu, C.J., Liu, S., & Willett, W.C. (2011). Informing food choices and health outcomes by use of the dietary glycemic index. *Nutr. Rev*, 69(4), 231–42.

15. Holt, S.H., Miller, J.C., Petocz, P., & Farmakalidis, E. (1995). A satiety index of common foods. *Eur J Clin Nutr*, 49(9), 675-90.

16. McCarrison, R. (1926). A Good Diet and a Bad One: An Experimental Contrast. *Br Med J*, 2(3433), 724-732.

17. Anderson, J. W., Baird, P., Davis, R. H. Jr, Ferreri, S., Knudtson, M., Koraym, A., Waters, V., Williams, C. L. (2009). Health benefits of dietary fiber. *Nutrition Reviews*, 67(4), 188-205.

18. Givens, D.I. (2010). Milk and meat in our diet: good or bad for health? *Animal*, 4(12), 1941-52.

19. Liu, P., Holman, C.D., Jin, J., & Zhang, M. (2015). Diet and risk of adult leukemia: a multicenter case-control study in China. *Cancer Causes Control*, 26(8), 1141-51.

20. Yamagishi, K., Iso, H., & Tsugane, S. (2015). Saturated fat intake and cardiovascular disease in Japanese population. *J Atheroscler Thromb*, 22(5), 435-9.

21. Abrams, H. L. (1980). *Journal of Applied Nutrition*, 32(2), 70-71.

22. Cheraskin, E. (1978). *Journal of Orthomolecular Psychiatry*, 7, 150-155.

23. Pitskhelauri, G. Z. (1982). *The Longest Living of Soviet Georgia*. New York: Human Sciences Press.

24. Kang-Jey, H. (1971). *Archeological Pathology*, 91, 387.

25. Mann, G. V. (1972). *American Journal of Epidemiology*, 95, 26-37.

26. Franklyn, D. (1996). The Healthiest Women in the World. *Health*, 57-63.

27. Abrams, H. L. (1980). *Journal of Applied Nutrition*, 32(2), 70-71.

28. Rackis, J. J. (1985). Qualitative Plant Foods in Human Nutrition, 35, 225.

29. Dhaka, V., Gulia, N., Ahlawat, K.S., & Khatkar, B.S. (2011). Trans fats—sources, health risks and alternative approach - A review. *J Food Sci Technol*, 48(5), 534-41.

30. Erasmus, U. (1993). *Fats that heal, fats that kill: The complete guide to fats, oils, cholesterol and human health*. Summertown (TN): Alive Books.

31. Ng, C.Y., Leong, X.F., Masbah, N., Adam, S.K., Kamisah, Y., & Jaarin, K. (2014). Heated vegetable oils and cardiovascular disease risk factors. *Vascul Pharmacol*, 61(1), 1-9

32. Castelli, W. (1992). Archives of Internal Medicine, 152, 1371-2.

33. Nutrition Week. (1991, March 22). 21,12:2-3

34. McGee, D.L. (1984). Ten year incidence of coronary heart disease in Honolulu Heart Programme — Relationship to nutrient intake. *Am J Epidemiol*, 119, 667-676.

35. Enig, & Mary, G. (1978). Federation Proceedings, 37(9), 2215-2220.

36. Cohen, A. (1963). *American Heart Journal*, 65, 291.

37. Plat. J. (2001). Oxidized plant sterols in human serum and lipid infusions as measured by combined gas-liquid chromatography-mass spectrometry. *J Lipid Res*, 42, 2030-2038.

38. Blaylock, R. (1997). *Excitotoxins: The taste that kills.* Santa Fe: Health Press.

39. Alpert, M. E., Hutt, M. S., Wogan, G. N., & Davidson, C. S. (1971). Association between aflatoxin content of food and hepatoma frequency in Uganda. *Cancer,* 28(1), 253–60.

40. Carnaghan, R. B. (1967). Hepatic tumours and other chronic liver changes in rats following a single oral administration of aflatoxin. *British Journal of Cancer,* 21(4), 811–14.

41. Young, R. (2000). *Sick and tired? Reclaim your inner terrain.* Woodland Publishing.

42. Chen, F., Cole, P., Mi, Z., & Xing, L. Y. (1993). Corn and wheat-flour consumption and mortality from esophageal cancer in Shanxi, China. *International Journal of Cancer,* 53(6), 902–6.

43. La Vecchia, C., Negri, E., Decarli, A., D'Avanzo. B., & Franceschi, S. (1987). A case-control study of diet and gastric cancer in Northern Italy. *International Journal of Cancer,* 40(4), 484–89.

44. Toth, B., Patil, K., Pyysalo, H., Stessman, C., & Gannett, P. (1992). Cancer induction in mice by feeding the raw false morel mushroom Gyromitra esculenta. *Cancer Research,* 52(8), 2279–84.

45. Ghadirian P. (1987). Thermal irritation and esophageal cancer in northern Iran. *Cancer,* 60(8), 1909–14.

46. Ingram, D. M., Nottage, E., & Roberts, T. (1991). The Role of Saccharomyces cerevisiae—baker's, or brewer's, yeast—in the development of breast cancer: A case control study of patients with breast cancer, benign epithelial hyperplasia and fibrocystic disease of the breast. *British Journal of Cancer,* 64(1), 187–91.

47. Stitt, P. (1981). *Fighting the Food Giants.* Natural Press, Manitowoc, WI.

48. Jenkins, D. (1981). *American Journal of Clinical Nutrition,* 34, 362-366.

49. Xiao, C.W. (2008). Health effects of soy protein and isoflavones in humans. *J Nutr,* 138(6), 1244S-9S.

50. D'Adamo, C.R., & Sahin, A. (2014). Soy foods and supplementation: a review of commonly perceived health benefits and risks. *Altern Ther Health Med,* 20(1), 39-51.

51. Trock, B.J., Hilakivi-Clarke, L., & Clarke, R. (2006). Meta-analysis of soy intake and breast cancer risk. *J Natl Cancer Inst,* 98(7), 459-71.

52. Allred, C.D. (2001). Soy diets containing varying amounts of genistein stimulate growth of estrogen-dependent

(MCF-7) tumors in a dose-dependent manner. *Cancer Res,* 61(13), 5045-50.

53. Tombak, M. (2006*). Cure the incurable.* Blaine. (WA): Healthy Life Press Inc.

54. Room, R., Babor, T., & Rehm, J. (2005). Alcohol and public health. *The Lancet,* 365(9458), 519–30.

55. Pöschl, G., & Seitz, H. K. (2004). Alcohol and cancer. *Alcohol and Alcoholism,* 39(3), 155–65.

56. Allen, N. E. (2009). Moderate alcohol intake and cancer incidence in women. *Journal of the National Cancer Institute,* 101(5), 296–305.

57. Mørch, L. S. (2007). Alcohol drinking, consumption patterns and breast cancer among Danish nurses: A cohort study. *European Journal of Public Health,* 17(6), 624–29.

58. Vartanian, L.R., Schwartz, M.B., & Brownell, K.D. (2007, February 28). Effects of soft drink consumption on nutrition and health: a systematic review and meta-analysis. *Am J Public Health,* 97(4), 667-75.

59. Fagherazzi, G., Vilier, A., Saes, S.D., Lajous, M., Balkau, B., Clavel-Chapelon, F. (2013). Consumption of artificially and sugar-sweetened beverages and incident type 2 diabetes in the Etude Epidemiologique aupres des femmes de la Mutuelle Generale de l'Education Nationale-European Prospective Investigation into Cancer and Nutrition cohort. *Am J Clin Nutr,* 97(3), 517-23.

60. Fowler, S.P., Williams, K., & Hazuda, H.P. (2015). Diet soda intake is associated with long-term increases in waist circumference in a biethnic cohort of older adults: the San Antonio Longitudinal Study of Aging. *J Am Geriatr Soc,* 63(4), 708-15.

61. Fowler, S.P., Williams, K., Resendez, R.G., Hunt, K.J., Hazuda, H.P., & Stern MP. (2008). Fueling the obesity epidemic? Artificially sweetened beverage use and long-term weight gain. *Obesity (Silver Spring, Md.)*, 16, 1894–1900.

62. Stellman, S.D., Garfinkel, L. (1986). Artificial sweetener use and one-year weight change among women. *Prev Med*, 15, 195–202.

63. Colditz, G.A., Willett, W.C., Stampfer, M.J., London, S.J., Segal, M.R., & Speizer, F.E. (1990). Patterns of weight change and their relation to diet in a cohort of healthy women. *Am J Clin Nutr*, 51, 1100–1105.

64. Striegel-Moore, R.H., Thompson, D., Affenito, S.G., Franko, D.L., Obarzanek, E., & Barton, B.A. (2006). Correlates of beverage intake in adolescent girls: the National Heart, Lung, and Blood Institute Growth and Health Study. *J Pediatr*, 148, 183–187.

65. Furth, A., & Harding, J. (1989). Why sugar is bad for you. *New Scientist*, 44.

66. Szanto, S., & Yudkin, J. (1969). The Effect of Dietary Sucrose on Blood Lipids, Serum Insulin, Platelet Adhesiveness and Body Weight in Human Volunteers. *Postgraduate Medicine Journal*, 45(527), 602–7.

67. Takahashi, E. (1982). Tohoku University School of Medicine. Wholistic Health Digest, 41.

68. Quillin, P. (2000). Cancer's Sweet Tooth. *Nutrition Science News*.

69. Michaud, D. (2002). Dietary sugar, glycemic load, and pancreatic cancer risk in a prospective study. *Journal of the National Cancer Institute*, 94(17), 1293–300.

70. Moerman, C. J. (1993). Dietary sugar intake in the aetiology of biliary tract cancer. *International Journal of Epidemiology*, 2(2), 207–14.

71. De Stefani, E. (1998). Dietary sugar and lung cancer: A case–control study in Uruguay. *Nutrition and Cancer*, 31(2), 132–37.

72. Cornée, J. (1995). A case-control study of gastric cancer and nutritional factors in Marseille, France. *European Journal of Epidemiology*, 11(1), 55–65.

73. Darlington, L., Ramsey, N. W., & Mansfield, J. R. (1986). Placebo-controlled, blind study of dietary manipulation therapy in rheumatoid arthritis. *The Lancet*, 8475(1), 236–38.

74. Erlander, S. (1979). The Cause and Cure of Multiple Sclerosis. *The Disease to End Disease*, 1(3), 59–63.

75. Beck, Nielsen, H., Pedersen O., & Schwartz, S.N. (1978). Effects of diet on the cellular insulin binding and the insulin sensitivity in young healthy subjects. *Diabetologia*, 15(4), 289-296.

76. Reiser, S. (1986). Effects of sugars on indices on glucose tolerance in humans. *American Journal of Clinical Nutrition*. 43(1), 151–59.

77. Tjäderhane, L., & Larmas, M. (1998). A high sucrose diet decreases the mechanical strength of bones in growing rats. *Journal of Nutrition*, 128(10), 1807–10.

78. Frey, J. (2001). Is there sugar in the Alzheimer's disease? *Annales de Biologie Clinique*, 59(3), 253–57.

79. Veromann, S. (2003). Dietary sugar and salt represent real risk factors for cataract development. *Ophthalmologica*, 217(4), 302–7.

80. Yudkin, J., Kang, S., & Bruckdorfer, K. (1980). Effects of high dietary sugar. *British Journal of Medicine*, 282(6259), 223–24.

81. Lechin, F. (1992). Effects of an oral glucose load on plasma neurotransmitters in humans: Involvement of REM sleep? *Neurophychobiology*, 26(1-2), 4–11.

82. Soffritti, M. (2010). Aspartame administered in feed, beginning prenatally through life span, induces cancers of the liver and lung in male Swiss mice. *American Journal of Industrial Medicine*, 53(12), 1197–206.

83. Inness-Brown, V. (2010). *My Aspartame Experiment: Report from a Private Citizen*. North Charleston (SC): BookSurge Publishing.

84. Potenza, D. P., & el-Mallakh, R. S. (1989). Aspartame: clinical update. *Connecticut Medicine*, 53(7), 395–400.

85. Swithers, S.E. (2013). Artificial sweeteners produce the counterintuitive effect of inducing metabolic derangements. *Trends Endocrinol Metab*, 24(9), 431-41.

86. Hampton T. (2008). Sugar substitutes linked to weight gain. *JAMA*. 299, 2137–8.

87. Laska, M.N. (2012). Longitudinal associations between key dietary behaviors and weight gain over time: transitions through the adolescent years. *Obesity (Silver Spring)*, 20, 118–125.

88. Tandel, K.R. (2011). Sugar substitutes: Health controversy over perceived benefits. *J Pharmacol Pharmacother*, 2(4), 236-43.

89. Goyal, S. K., Samsher, Goyal, R. K. (2010). Stevia (Stevia rebaudiana) a bio-sweetener: a review. *International Journal of Food Sciences and Nutrition*, 61(1), 1–10.

90. Lailerd, N., Saengsirisuwan, V., Sloniger, J.A., Toskulkao, C., & Henriksen, E. J. (2004). Effects of stevioside on glucose transport activity in insulin-sensitive and insulin-resistant rat skeletal muscle. *Metabolism—Clinical and Experimental*, 53(1), 101–7.

91. Jeppesen, P. B. (2003). Antihyperglycemic and blood pressure-reducing effects of stevioside in the diabetic Goto-Kakizaki rat. *Metabolism Clinical and Experimental*, 52(3), 372–78.

92. Dyrskog, S. E., Jeppesen, P. B., Colombo, M., Abudula, R., & Hermansen, K. (2005). Preventive effects of a soy-based diet supplemented with stevioside on the development of the metabolic syndrome and type 2 diabetes in Zucker diabetic fatty rats. *Metabolism Clinical and Experimental*, 54(9), 1181–88.

93. Jones, R. (2001). *Honey and healing through the ages.* InP. Munn, & R. Jones (Eds.), Honey and Healing. Cardiff: International Bee Research Association.

94. Marcucci M. C. (1995). Propolis: chemical composition, biological properties and therapeutical activity. *Apidologie*, 26(2), 83–99.

95. Castaldo, S., & Capasso, F. (2002). Propolis, an old remedy used in modern medicine. *Fitoterapia*, 73(Suppl 1), S1–6. Molan, P. C. (1999). Why honey is effective as a medicine. 1. Its use in modern medicine. *Bee World*, 80(2), 80–92.

96. Manyi-Loh, C. E., Clarke, A. M., & Ndip, R. N. (2011). An overview of honey: Therapeutic properties and contribution in nutrition and human health. *African Journal of Microbiology Research*, 5(8), 844–52.

97. Buratti, S., Benedetti, S., & Cosio, M. S. (2007). Evaluation of the antioxidant power of honey, propolis and royal

jelly by amperometric flow injection analysis. *Talanta, 71(3)*, 1387–92.

98. Bogdanov, S. (2011). Functional and Biological Properties of the Bee Products: a Review. *Bee Product Science online*. Retrieved from www.bee-hexagon.net, 1-12.

99. Tamura, T., Fujii, A., Kuboyama, N. (1987). Anti-tumor effects of royal jelly (RJ). *Nippon Yakurigaku Zasshi, 89(2)*, 73–80.

100. Nakaya, M., Onda, H., Sasaki, K., Yukiyoshi, A., Tachibana, H., & Yamada, K. (2007). Effect of royal jelly on bisphenol A-induced proliferation of human breast cancer cells. *Bioscience, Biotechnology and Biochemistry, 71(1)*, 253–55.

101. Oršolić, N., Sacases, F., Percie du Sert, P., & Bašić, I. (2007). Antimetastatic ability of honey bee products. *Periodicum Biologorum, 109(2)*, 173–80.

102. Mavric, E., Wittman, S., Barth, G., & Henle, T. (2008). Identification and quantification of methylglyoxal as the dominant antibacterial constituent of Manuka (Leptospermum scoparium) honeys from New Zealand. *Molecular Nutrition and Food Research, 52(4)*, 483–89.

103. Nagai, T., Sakai, M., Inoue, R., Inoue, H., & Suzuki, N. (2001). Antioxidative activities of some commercially honeys, royal jelly, and propolis. *Food Chemistry, 75(2)*, 237–40.

104. Kimura, M., & Itokawa, Y. (1990). Cooking losses of minerals in foods and its nutritional significance. *Journal of Nutritional Science and Vitaminology, 36(Suppl 1)* S25–32, S33.

105. Adzersen, K. H., Jess, P., Freivogel, K. W., Gerhard, I., & Bastert, G. (2003). Raw and cooked vegetables, fruits,

selected micronutrients, and breast cancer risk: A case-control study in Germany. *Nutrition and Cancer,* 46(2), 131–37.

106. Yuan, G. F., Sun, B., Yuan, J., & Wang, Q. M. (2009). Effects of different cooking methods on health-promoting compounds of broccoli. *Journal of Zhejiang University Science,* 10(8), 580–88.

107. Jägerstad, M., & Skog, K. (2005). Genotoxicity of heat-processed foods. *Mutation Research,* 574(1-2), 156–72.

108. Cross, A, J. (2010). A large prospective study of meat consumption and colorectal cancer risk: An investigation of potential mechanisms underlying this association. *Cancer Research,* 70(6), 2406–14.

109. Anderson, K, E. (2002). Meat intake and cooking techniques: Associations with pancreatic cancer. *Mutation Research,* 506-7, 225–31.

200. Stolzenberg-Solomon, R. Z. (2007). Meat and meat-mutagen intake and pancreatic cancer risk in the NIH-AARP cohort. *Cancer Epidemiology, Biomarkers, and Prevention,* 16(12), 2664–75.

201. Carlsen, M. H. (2010). The total antioxidant content of more than 3100 foods, beverages, spices, herbs and supplements used worldwide. *Nutrition Journal,* 9.

202. Katz, D.L., Doughty, K., & Ali, A. (2011). Cocoa and chocolate in human health and disease. *Antioxid Redox Signal,* 15(10), 2779-811.

203. Yuan, G.F., Sun, B., Yuan, J., & Wang, Q.M. (2009). Effects of different cooking methods on health-promoting compounds of broccoli. *J Zhejiang Univ Sci B,* 10(8), 580-8.

204. López-Berenguer, C., Carvajal, M., Moreno, D.A., & García-Viguera, C. (2007). Effects of microwave cooking conditions on bioactive compounds present in broccoli inflorescences. *J Agric Food Chem,* 55(24), 10001-7.

205. Taghavi, N., & Yazdi, I. (2007). Type of food and risk of oral cancer. *Arch Iran Med,* 10(2), 227-32.

206. Rupérez, P. (2002). Mineral content of edible marine seaweeds. *Food Chemistry,* 79(1), 23–26.

207. Teas, J. (1983). The dietary intake of Laminaria, a brown seaweed, and breast cancer prevention. *Nutrition and Cancer,* 4(3), 217–22.

208. Tokudome, S., Kuriki, K., & Moore, M. A. (2001). Seaweed and Cancer Prevention. *Japanese Journal of Cancer Research,* 92(9), 1008–10.

209. Yuan, Y. V., & Walsh, N. A. (2006). Antioxidant and antiproliferative activities of extracts from a variety of edible seaweeds. *Food and Chemical Toxicology,* 44(7), 1144–50.

210. Teas, J., Harbison, M. L., & Gelman, R. S. (1984). Dietary seaweed (Laminaria) and mammary carcinogenesis in rats. *Cancer Research,* 44(7), 2758–61.

211. Cho, E. J., Rhee, S. H., & Park, K. Y. (1998). Antimutagenic and cancer cell growth inhibitory effects of seaweeds. *Journal of Food Science and Nutrition,* 2(4), 348–53.

212. Funahashi, H. (2001). Seaweed prevents breast cancer? *Japanese Journal of Cancer Research,* 92(5), 483–87.

213. Trudeau, K. (2005). *Natural Cures "They" Don't Want You To Know About.* Elk Groove Village (IL): Alliance Publishing.

214. Saleh, M.A. (1980). Mutagenic and carcinogenic effects of pesticides. *J Environ Sci Health B,* 15(6), 907-27.

215. Di Renzo, L. (2007). Is antioxidant plasma status in humans a consequence of the antioxidant food content influence? *European Review for Medical and Pharmacological Sciences,* 11(3), 185–92.

216. Benbrook, C., Zhao, X., Yáñez, J., Davies, N., & Andrews, P. (2008). New evidence confirms the nutritional superiority of plant-based organic foods. *The Organic Center Publication.*

217. Worthington, V. (2001). Nutritional quality of organic versus conventional fruits, vegetables and grains. *Journal of Alternative and Complementary Medicine,* 7(2), 161–73.

218. Woese, K., Lange, D., Boess, C., & Bögl, K. W. (1997). A comparison of organically and conventionally grown foods—results of a review of the relevant literature. *Journal of the Science of Food and Agriculture,* 74(3), 281–93.

219. Juchimiuk, J., Gnys, A., & Maluszynska, J. (2006). DNA damage induced by mutagens in plant and human cell nuclei in acellular comet assay. *Folia Histochem Cytobiol,* 44(2), 127-31.

220. Ponnampalam, R., Mondy, N.I., & Babish, J.G. (1983). A review of environmental and health risks of maleic hydrazide. *Regul Toxicol Pharmacol,* 3(1), 38-47.

221. Sandhu, S.S., & Waters, M.D. (1980). Mutagenicity evaluation of chemical pesticides. *J Environ Sci Health B,* 15(6), 929-48.

222. Swietlińska, Z., & Zuk, J. (1978). Cytotoxic effects of maleic hydrazide. *Mutat Res,* 55(1), 15-30.

223. Haenlein, G. F. W. (2004). Goat milk in human nutrition. *Small Ruminant Research,* 51(2), 155–63.

224. Morales, E. (2005). Nutritional value of goat and cow milk protein. *Options Méditerranéennes, Series A,* (67), 167–70.

225. Yosef, S., & Reuven, Y. (2005). Etiology of autism and camel milk as therapy.□*International Journal on Disability and Human Development,* 4(2), 67-70.

226. Agrawal, R.P., Beniwal, R., Sharma, S., Kochar, D.K., Tuteja, F.C., Ghorui, S.K., & Sahani, M.S. (2005). Effect of raw camel milk in type 1 diabetic patients: 1 year randomised study. □*Journal of Camel Practice and Research,* 12(1), 27-35.

227. Yosef, S., Reuben, B., Mark, M., & Reuven, Y. (2005). Camel milk for food allergies in children. *Isr Med Assoc J,* 7(12), 796-8.

228. Matthews, J. (2011, November 15). *Camel Milk: Healing or Hype?* Retrieved from http://nourishinghope.com/2011/11/camel-milk-healing-or-hype/

229. Nikkhah, A. (2011). Science of Camel and Yak Milks: Human Nutrition and Health Perspectives. *Food and Nutrition Sciences,* 2(6), 2011, 667-673.

230. Foekel, C., Schubert, R., & Kaatz, M. (2009). Dietetic effects of oral intervention with mare's milk on the Severity Scoring of Atopic Dermatitis, on faecal microbiota and on immunological parameters in patients with atopic dermatitis. *Int J Food Sci Nutr,* 60 Suppl 7, 41-52.

231. Abdel-Salam, A.M., Al-Dekheil, A., Babkr, A., Farahna, M., & Mousa, H.M. (2010). High fiber probiotic

fermented mare's milk reduces the toxic effects of mercury in rats. *N Am J Med Sci,* 2(12), 569-75.

232. Jirillo, F., Jirillo, E., & Magrone, T. (2010). Donkey's and goat's milk consumption and benefits to human health with special reference to the inflammatory status. *Curr Pharm Des,* 16(7), 859-63.

233. Theodoulou, M. (2014, December 26). *Could DONKEY MILK be the elixir of life? You can drink it - or even wash with it, like Cleopatra. Why experts say asses' milk may have remarkable anti-ageing powers.* Retrieved from http://www.dailymail.co.uk/health/article-2887306/Could-DONKEY-MILK-elixir-life.html

234. Guo, X., Long, R., & Kreuzer, M. (2014). Importance of functional ingredients in yak milk-derived food on health of Tibetan nomads living under high-altitude stress: a review. *Crit Rev Food Sci Nutr,* 54(3), 292-302.

235. Crewe, J. (1929). Raw milk cures many diseases. *Certified Milk Magazine,* 3–6.

236. Gordon, W. (2009, June 2). Raw milk seen as an important part of natural-cancer-therapy-protocol. *The Bovine.*

237. Ramiel, N., & George, W. H. *Raw Milk Beats Tooth Decay.*

238. Mattick, E., & Golding, J. (1931). Relative value of raw and heated milk in nutrition. *The Lancet,* 217(5612), 662–67.

239. Melnik, B. C. (2015). The pathogenic role of persistent milk signaling in mTORC1- and milk-microRNA-driven type 2 diabetes mellitus. *Curr Diabetes Rev,* 11(1), 46-62.

240. Ponnampalam, E.N., Mann, N.J., & Sinclair, A.J. (2006). Effect of feeding systems on omega-3 fatty acids, conjugated linoleic acid and trans fatty acids in Australian

beef cuts: potential impact on human health. *Asia Pac J Clin Nutr,* 15(1), 21-9.

241. Leaf, A. (2007). Prevention of sudden cardiac death by n-3 polyunsaturated fatty acids. *J Cardiovasc Med. (Hagerstown),* 8 Suppl 1, S27-29.

242. Dhiman, T. R., & Anand.G.R. (1999). Conjugated linoleic acid content of milk from cows fed different diets. *J Dairy Sci,* 82(10), 2146-56.

243. Damson, R.H. (1990) Mutagens and carcinogens formed during cooking of foods and methods to minimize their formation. *Cancer Prevention,* 1-7.

244. Sugimura, T., Wakabayashi, K., Nakagama, H., & Nagao, M. (2004). Heterocyclic amines: Mutagens/carcinogens produced during cooking of meat and fish. *Cancer Science,* 95(4), 290-299.

245. Cross, A.J., Ferrucci, L.M., & Risch, A. (2010). A large prospective study of meat consumption and colorectal cancer risk: An investigation of potential mechanisms underlying this association. *Cancer Research,* 70(6), 2406–2414.

246. Anderson, K.E., Sinha, R., & Kulldorff, M. (2002). Meat intake and cooking techniques: Associations with pancreatic cancer. *Mutation Research,* 506–507, 225–231.

247. Stolzenberg-Solomon, R.Z., Cross, A.J., & Silverman, D.T. (2007). Meat and meat-mutagen intake and pancreatic cancer risk in the NIH-AARP cohort. *Cancer Epidemiology, Biomarkers, and Prevention,* 16(12), 2664–2675.

248. Cross, A.J., Peters, U., & Kirsh, V.A. (2005). A prospective study of meat and meat mutagens and prostate cancer risk. *Cancer Research,* 65(24), 11779–11784.

249. Sinha, R., Park, Y., & Graubard, B.I. (2009). Meat and meat-related compounds and risk of prostate cancer in a large

prospective cohort study in the United States. *American Journal of Epidemiology,* 170(9), 1165–1177.

250. Habermeyer, M., Roth, A., & Guth, S. (2015). Nitrate and nitrite in the diet: how to assess their benefit and risk for human health. *Mol Nutr Food Res,* 59(1), 106-28.

251. Karsten, H.D., Patterson, P.H., Stout, R., & Crews, G. (2010). Vitamins A, E and fatty acid composition of the eggs of caged hens and pastured hens. Renew. Agric. *Food Syst,* 25, 45–54.

252. Lopez-Bote, C. J., Sanz, R., Arias, A.I., Rey, A., Castano, B., & Isabel, J. (1998). Effect of free-range feeding on omega-3 fatty acids and alpha-tocopherol content and oxidative stability of eggs. *Animal Feed Science and Technology,* 72, 33-40.

253. Vander, W.J., Gupta, A., Khosla, P., & Dhurandhar, N.V. (2008). Egg breakfast enhances weight loss. *Int J Obes (Lond),* 32(10), 1545-51.

254. Cocoros, G., Cahn, P. H., & Siler, W. (1973). Mercury concentrations in fish, plankton and water from three Western Atlantic estuaries. *Journal of Fish Biology,* 5(6), 641–7.

255. Storelli, M. M., & Marcotrigiano, G. O. (2001). Total mercury levels in muscle tissue of swordfish (Xiphias gladius) and bluefin tuna (Thunnus thynnus) from the Mediterranean Sea (Italy). *Journal of Food Protection,* 64(7), 1058–61.

256. Jureša, D., & Blanuša, M. (2003). Mercury, arsenic, lead and cadmium in fish and shellfish from the Adriatic Sea. *Food Additives and Contaminants,* 20(3), 241–46.

257. Shaw, S. D., Brenner, D., Berger, M. L., Carpenter, D. O., Hong, C., & Kannan, K. (2006). PCBs, PCDD/Fs, and organochlorine pesticides in farmed Atlantic salmon from

Maine, eastern Canada, and Norway, and wild salmon from Alaska. *Environmental Science and Technology*, 40(17), 5347–54.

258. Easton, M. D., Luszniak, D., & Von der, G.E. (2002). Preliminary examination of contaminant loadings in farmed salmon, wild salmon and commercial salmon feed. *Chemosphere*, 46(7), 1053–74.

259. Hites, R. A., Foran, J. A., Carpenter, D. O., Hamilton, M. C., Knuth, B. A., & Schwager, S. J. (2004). Global assessment of organic contaminants in farmed salmon. *Science*, 303(5655), 226–29.

260. Hites, R. A., Foran, J. A., Schwager, S. J., Knuth, B. A., Hamilton, M. C., & Carpenter, D. O. (2004). Global assessment of polybrominated diphenyl ethers in farmed and wild salmon. *Environmental Science and Technology*, 38(19), 4945–49.

261. Airey, D. (1983). Total mercury concentrations in human hair from 13 countries in relation to fish consumption and location. *Science of the Total Environment*, 31(2), 157–80.

262. Mozaffarian, D., & Rimm, E. B. (2006). Fish intake, contaminants, and human health: evaluating the risks and the benefits. *Journal of the American Medical Association*, 296(15), 1885–99.

263. Dougherty, C.P., Henricks, H.S., & Reinert, J.C. (2000). Dietary exposures to food contaminants across the United States. *Environ Res*, 84(2), 170-85.

264. Lyche, J.L., Rosseland, C., Berge, G., & Polder, A. (2015). Human health risk associated with brominated flame-retardants (BFRs). *Environ Int*, 74, 170-80.

265. Mattes, R.D., Kris-Etherton, P.M., & Foster, G.D. (2008). Impact of peanuts and tree nuts on body weight and healthy weight loss in adults. *J Nutr,* 138(9), 1741S-1745S.

266. Mattes, R.D., & Dreher, M.L. (2010). Nuts and healthy body weight maintenance mechanisms. *Asia Pac J Clin Nutr,* 19(1), 137-41.

267. Mattes, R.D. (2008). The energetics of nut consumption. *Asia Pac J Clin Nutr,* 17, Suppl 1, 337-9.

268. Claesson, A.L., Holm, G., Ernersson, A., Lindström, T., Nystrom, F.H. (2009). Two weeks of overfeeding with candy, but not peanuts, increases insulin levels and body weight. *Scand J Clin Lab Invest,* 69(5), 598-605.

269. Reis, C.E., Ribeiro, D.N., Costa, N.M., Bressan, J., Alfenas, R.C., & Mattes, R.D. (2013). Acute and second-meal effects of peanuts on glycaemic response and appetite in obese women with high type 2 diabetes risk: a randomised cross-over clinical trial. *Br J Nutr,* 109(11), 2015-23.

270. Hu, F.B., & Willett W.C. (2002). Optimal diets for prevention of coronary heart disease. *J. Am. Med. Assoc,* 288, 2569–2578.

271. Ros, E. (2010). Health benefits of nut consumption. *Nutrients,* 2(7), 652-82.

272. Slavin, J. (2004). Whole grains and human health. *Nutr Res Rev,* 17(1), 99-110.

273. Rajasree P, R., & Raghesh, V. (2006). Health Benefits Of Whole Grains: A Literature Review. *The Internet Journal of Nutrition and Wellness,* 4, 2.

274. Ferruzzi, M.G., Jonnalagadda, S.S., & Liu, S. (2014, March 1). Developing a standard definition of whole-grain foods for dietary recommendations: summary report of a

multidisciplinary expert roundtable discussion. *Adv Nutr,* 5(2), 164-76.

275. Okarter, N., Liu, R.H. (2010). Health benefits of whole grain phytochemicals. *Crit Rev Food Sci Nutr.* 50(3), 193-208.

278. Belobrajdic, D.P., & Bird, A.R. (2013). The potential role of phytochemicals in wholegrain cereals for the prevention of type-2 diabetes. *Nutr J,* 12, 62.

279. Slavin, J. (2003). Why whole grains are protective: biological mechanisms. *Proc Nutr Soc,* 62(1), 129-34.

280. Mudryj, A.N., Yu, N., & Aukema, H.M. (2014). Nutritional and health benefits of pulses. *Appl Physiol Nutr Metab,* 39(11), 1197-204.

281. Jonnalagadda, S.S., Harnack, L., Liu, R.H., McKeown, N., Seal, C., Liu, S., Fahey, G.C. (2011). Putting the whole grain puzzle together: health benefits associated with whole grains--summary of American Society for Nutrition 2010 Satellite Symposium. J Nutr, 141(5), 1011S-22S.

282. Reinhold, J.G. (1972). Ecology of Food and Nutrition, 1, 187-192.

283. Dixit, A.A., Azar, K.M., Gardner, C.D., & Palaniappan, L.P. (2011). Incorporation of whole, ancient grains into a modern Asian Indian diet to reduce the burden of chronic disease. *Nutr Rev,* 69(8), 479-88.

284. Bressani, R., de Martell, E.C., & de Godínez, C.M. (1993). Protein quality evaluation of amaranth in adult humans. *Plant Foods Hum Nutr,* 43(2), 123-43.

285. Miller, J.B., Pang, E., & Bramall, L. (1992). Rice: a high or low glycemic index food? *Am J Clin Nutr,* 56(6), 1034-6.

286. Fitzgerald, M. (2012). Identification of a major genetic determinant of glycaemic index in rice. *Rice*, 4(2), 66-74.

287. Trinidad, T.P., Mallillin, A.C., Encabo, R.R., Sagum, R.S., Felix, A.D., & Juliano, B.O. (2013). The effect of apparent amylose content and dietary fibre on the glycemic response of different varieties of cooked milled and brown rice. *Int J Food Sci Nutr*, 64(1), 89-93.

288. Ranawana, D.V., Henry, C.J., Lightowler, H.J., & Wang, D. (2009). Glycaemic index of some commercially available rice and rice products in Great Britain. *Int J Food Sci Nutr*, 60 Suppl 4, 99-110.

289. Kataoka, M., Venn, B.J., Williams, S.M., Morenga, L.A., Heemels, I.M., & Mann, J.I. (2013). Glycaemic responses to glucose and rice in people of Chinese and European ethnicity. *Diabet Med*, 30(3), e101-7.

290. Atkinson, F.S., Foster-Powell, K.,& Brand-Miller, J.C. (2008). International tables of glycemic index and glycemic load values: 2008. *Diabetes Care*, 31(12), 2281-3.

291. Maioli, M., Pes, G.M., Sanna, M., Cherchi, S., Dettori, M., Manca, E., & Farris, G.A. (2008). Sourdough-leavened bread improves postprandial glucose and insulin plasma levels in subjects with impaired glucose tolerance. *Acta Diabetol*, 45(2), 91-6.

292. Greco, L., Gobbetti, M., & Auricchio, R. (2011). Safety for patients with celiac disease of baked goods made of wheat flour hydrolyzed during food processing. *Clin Gastroenterol Hepatol*, 9(1), 24-9.

293. Drisko, J., Giles, C.K., & Bischoff, B.J. (2003). Probiotics in health maintenance and disease prevention. *Altern Med Rev*, 8(2), 143-55.

294. Yan, F., & Polk, D.B. (2011). Probiotics and immune health. *Curr Opin Gastroenterol,* 27(6), 496-501.

295. Singh, V.P., Sharma, J., Babu, S., Rizwanulla, Singla, A. (2013). Role of probiotics in health and disease: a review. *J Pak Med Assoc,* 63(2):253-7.

296. Collado, M.C., Isolauri, E., Salminen, S., & Sanz, Y. (2009). The impact of probiotic on gut health. *Curr Drug Metab,* 10(1), 68-78.

297. Balakrishnan, M., Floch, M.H. (2012). Prebiotics, probiotics and digestive health. *Curr Opin Clin Nutr Metab Care,* 15(6), 580-5.

298. Gage, J. (2009). Understanding the role of probiotics in supporting digestive comfort. *Nurs Stand,* 24(4), 47-55.

299. Mohamed el-O, A., Mohamed, S.M., & Mohamed, K.A. (2001). The effect of cider vinegar on some nutritional and physiological parameters in mice. *J Egypt Public Health Assoc,* 76(1-2), 17-36.

300. Nazıroğlu, M., Güler, M., Özgül, C., Saydam, G., Küçükayaz, M., & Sözbir, E. (2014). Apple cider vinegar modulates serum lipid profile, erythrocyte, kidney, and liver membrane oxidative stress in ovariectomized mice fed high cholesterol. *J Membr Biol,* 247(8), 667-73.

301. Johnston, C.S., & Gaas, C.A. (2006). Vinegar: medicinal uses and antiglycemic effect. *MedGenMed,* 8(2), 61.

302. Gambon, D.L., Brand, H.S., & Veerman, E.C. (2012). [Unhealthy weight loss. Erosion by apple cider vinegar]. *Ned Tijdschr Tandheelkd,* 119(12), 589-91.

303. Okabe, S., Okamoto, T., Zhao, C.M., Chen, D., & Matsui, H. (2014). Acetic acid induces cell death: an in vitro study using normal rat gastric mucosal cell line and rat and

human gastric cancer and mesothelioma cell lines. *J Gastro-enterol Hepatol,* 29(4), 65-9.

304. Nishino, H., Murakoshi, M., & Mou, X.Y. (2005). Cancer prevention by phytochemicals. *Oncology,* 69(1), 38–40.

305. Nishidai, S., Nakamura, Y., & Torikai K. (2000). Kurosu, a traditional vinegar produced from unpolished rice, suppresses lipid peroxidation in vitro and in mouse skin. *Biosci Biotechnol Biochem,* 64, 1909–1914.

306. Rajaram, S. (2014). Health benefits of plant-derived α-linolenic acid. *Am J Clin Nutr,* 100(1), 443S-8S.

307. Stark, A.H., Crawford, M.A., & Reifen R. (2008). Update on alpha-linolenic acid. *Nutr Rev,* 66(6), 326-32.

308. Martinchik, A.N., Baturin, A.K., Zubtsov, V.V., & Molofeev, V. (2012). Nutritional value and functional properties of flaxseed. *Vopr Pitan,* 81(3), 4-10.

309. Kristensen, M., Savorani, F., & Christensen, S. (2013). Flaxseed dietary fibers suppress postprandial lipemia and appetite sensation in young men. *Nutr Metab Cardiovasc Dis,* 23(2), 136-43.

310. Ibrügger, S., Kristensen, M., Mikkelsen, M.S., & Astrup, A. (2012). Flaxseed dietary fiber supplements for suppression of appetite and food intake. *Appetite,* 58(2), 490-5.

311. Cassani, R.S., Fassini, P.G., Silvah, J.H., Lima, C.M., & Marchini, J.S. (2015). Impact of weight loss diet associated with flaxseed on inflammatory markers in men with cardiovascular risk factors: a clinical study. *Nutr J,* 14, 5.

312. Patade, A., Devareddy, L., Lucas, E.A., Korlagunta, K., Daggy, B.P., Arjmandi, B.H. (2008). Flaxseed reduces total and LDL cholesterol concentrations in Native American

postmenopausal women. *J Women's Health (Larchmt),* 17(3), 355-66.

313. Fukumitsu, S., Aida, K., Shimizu, H., & Toyoda, K. (2010). Flaxseed lignan lowers blood cholesterol and decreases liver disease risk factors in moderately hypercholesterolemic men. *Nutr Res,* 30(7), 441-6.

314. Bashir, S., Ali, S., & Khan, F. (2015). Partial Reversal of Obesity-Induced Insulin Resistance Owing to Anti-Inflammatory Immunomodulatory Potential of Flaxseed Oil. *Immunol Invest,* 44(5), 451-69.

315. Thakur, G., Mitra, A., Pal, K., & Rousseau, D. (2009). Effect of flaxseed gum on reduction of blood glucose and cholesterol in type 2 diabetic patients. *Int J Food Sci Nutr,* 60(6), 26-36.

316. Assunção, M.L., Ferreira, H.S., dos Santos, A.F., Cabral, C.R., Florêncio, T.M. (2009). Effects of dietary coconut oil on the biochemical and anthropometric profiles of women presenting abdominal obesity. *Lipids,* 44(7), 593-601.

317. Liau, K.M., Lee, Y.Y., Chen, C.K., Rasool, A.H. (2011). An open-label pilot study to assess the efficacy and safety of virgin coconut oil in reducing visceral adiposity. *ISRN Pharmacol,* 949686.

318. Maury, W., Price, J.P., & Brindley, M.A. (2009). Identification of light-independent inhibition of human immunodeficiency virus-1 infection through bioguided fractionation of Hypericum perforatum. *Virol J,* 6, 101.

319. Nevin, K.G., & Rajamohan, T. (2004). Beneficial effects of virgin coconut oil on lipid parameters and in vitro LDL oxidation. *Clinical Biochemistry,* 37(9), 830–835.

320. Yeap, S.K., Beh, B.K., & Ali, N.M. (2015). Antistress and antioxidant effects of virgin coconut oil in vivo. *Exp Ther Med,* 9(1), 39-42.

321. St-Onge, M.P., & Bosarge, A. (2008). Weight-loss diet that includes consumption of medium-chain triacylglycerol oil leads to a greater rate of weight and fat mass loss than does olive oil. *Am J Clin Nutr,* 87(3), 621-6.

322. Hashim, S.A., Bergen, S.S., Krell, K., & Van Itallie, T.B. (1964). Intestinal absorption and mode of transport in portal vein of medium chain fatty acids. *Journal of Clinical Investigation,* 43, 1238.

323. Yang, C. S., & Landau, J. M. (2000). Effects of tea consumption on nutrition and health. *The Journal of Nutrition,* 130(10), 2409–12.

324. Vipin, K., Sharma, A., Bhattacharya, A., Kumar, Hitesh, & K. Sharma. (2007). Health benefits of tea Consumption. *Tropical Journal of Pharmaceutical Research,* 6(3), 785–92.

325. Rietveld, A., & Wiseman, S. (2003). Antioxidant effects of tea: Evidence from human clinical trials. *The Journal of Nutrition,* 133(10), 3285S–3292S.

326. Jankun, J., Selman, S. H., Swiercz, R., & Skrzypczak-Jankun, E. (1997). Why drinking green tea could prevent cancer. *Nature,* 387(6633), 561.

327. Katiyar, S. K., & Mukhtar, H. (1997). Tea antioxidants in cancer chemoprevention. *Journal of Cellular Biochemistry,* 27, S59–67.

328. Sinija, V. R., & Mishra, H. N. (2008). Green tea: Health benefits. *Journal of Nutritional and Environmental Medicine,* 17(4), 232–42.

329. Mason, R. (2001). 200 mg of Zen; L-theanine boosts alpha waves, promotes alert relaxation. *Alternative & Complementary Therapies,* 7(2), 91–95.

330. Nakachi, K., Matsuyama, S., Miyake, S., Suganuma, M., & Imai, K. (2000). Preventive effects of drinking green tea on cancer and cardiovascular disease: Epidemiological evidence for multiple targeting prevention. *Biofactors,* 13(1–4), 49–54.

331. Duh, P. D., Yen, G. C., Yen, W. J., Wang, B. S., & Chang, L. W. (2004). Effects of pu-erh tea on oxidative damage and nitric oxide scavenging. *Journal of Agricultural and Food Chemistry,* 52(26), 8169–76.

332. Gong, J. S., Peng, C. X., He, X., Li, J. H., Li, B. C., & Zhou, H. J. (2009). Antioxidant activity of extracts of pu-erh tea and its material. *Asian Journal of Agricultural Sciences,* 1(2), 48–54.

333. Santana-Rios, G. (2001). Potent antimutagenic activity of white tea in comparison with green tea in the Salmonella assay. *Mutation Research,* 495(1-2), 61–74.

34. Smith, A. (2002). Effects of caffeine on human behavior. *Food and Chemical Toxicology,* 40(9), 1243–55.

335. Lorist, M. M., Snel, J., Kok, A., & Mulder, G. (1994). Influence of caffeine on selective attention in well-rested and fatigued subjects. *Psychophysiology,* 31(6), 525-534.

336. Higdon, J. V., & Frei, B. (2006). Coffee and health: A review of recent human research. *Critical Reviews In Food Science and Nutrition,* 46(2), 101–23.

337. Butt, M. S., & Sultan, M. T. (2011). Coffee and its consumption: Benefits and risks. *Critical Reviews in Food Science and Nutrition,* 51(4), 363–73.

338. Klatsky, A.L., Morton, C., Udaltsova, N., & Friedman, G.D. (2006). Coffee, cirrhosis, and transaminase enzymes. *Archives of Internal Medicine*, 166(11), 1190–95.

339. Corrao, G., Zambon, A., Bagnardi, V., D'Amicis, A., & Klatsky, A. (2001). Coffee, caffeine, and the risk of liver cirrhosis. *Annals of Epidemiology*, 11(7), 458–65.

340. Zhang, Y., Lee, E. T., Cowan, L. D., Fabsitz, R. R., & Howard, B. V. (2011). Coffee consumption and the incidence of type 2 diabetes in men and women with normal glucose tolerance: The Strong Heart Study. *Nutrition, Metabolism and Cardiovascular Diseases,* 21(6), 418–23.

341. Shimazu, T. (2005). Coffee consumption and the risk of primary liver cancer: Pooled analysis of two prospective studies in Japan. *International Journal of Cancer*, 116(1), 150–54.

342. Li, J., Seibold, P. (2011). Coffee consumption modifies risk of estrogen-receptor negative breast cancer. *Breast Cancer Research*, 13(3), R49.

343. Yu, X., Bao, Z., Zou, J., & Dong, J. (2011). Coffee consumption and risk of cancers: A meta-analysis of cohort studies. *BMC Cancer*, 11, 96.

344. Je, Y., & Giovannucci, E. (2011). Coffee consumption and risk of endometrial cancer: Findings from a large up-to-date meta-analysis. *International Journal of Cancer*, 131(7), 1700-10.

345. Je, Y., Hankinson, S. E., Tworoger, S. S., Devivo, I., & Giovannucci, E. (2011). A prospective cohort study of coffee consumption and risk of endometrial cancer over a 26-year follow-up. *Cancer Epidemiology, Biomarkers and Prevention*, 20(12), 2487–95.

346. Hamer, M. (2006). Coffee and health: Explaining conflicting results in hypertension. *Journal of Human Hypertension,* 20(12), 909–12.

347. Andersen, L. F., Jacobs Jr., D. R., Carlsen, M. H., & Blomhoff, R. (2006). Consumption of coffee is associated with reduced risk of death attributed to inflammatory and cardiovascular diseases in the Iowa Women's Health Study. *The American Journal of Clinical Nutrition,* 83(5), 1039–46.

348. Floegel, A., Pischon, T., Bergmann, M. M., Teucher, B., Kaaks, R., & Boeing, H. (2012). Coffee consumption and risk of chronic disease in the European Prospective Investigation into Cancer and Nutrition (EPIC)—Germany study. *The American Journal of Clinical Nutrition,* 95(4), 901–8.

349. Ames, B. N., & Gold, L. S. (1998). The causes and prevention of cancer: the role of environment. *Biotherapy,* 11(2–3), 205–20.

350. Janssens, P.L., Hursel, R., Martens, E.A., & Westerterp-Plantenga, M.S. (2013). Acute effects of capsaicin on energy expenditure and fat oxidation in negative energy balance. *PLoS One,* 8(7), e67786.

351. Aggarwal, B.B., Sundaram, C., Malani, N., & Ichikawa, H. (2007). Curcumin: the Indian solid gold. *Adv Exp Med Biol,* 595, 1-75.

352. Lagouri, V., & Boskou, D. (1996). Nutrient antioxidants in oregano. *Int J Food Sci Nutr,* 47(6), 493-7.

353. Zheng, W., & Wang, S.Y. (2001). Antioxidant activity and phenolic compounds in selected herbs. *J Agric Food Chem,* 49(11), 5165-70.

354. Savini, I., Arnone, R., Catani, M.V., & Avigliano, L. (2009). Origanum vulgare induces apoptosis in human colon cancer caco2 cells. *Nutr Cancer,* 61(3), 381-9.

355. Allen, R.W., Schwartzman, E., Baker, W.L., Coleman, C.I., & Phung, O.J. (2013). Cinnamon use in type 2 diabetes: an updated systematic review and meta-analysis. *Ann Fam Med,* 11(5), 452-9.

356. Dhandapani, S., Subramanian, V.R., Rajagopal, S., & Namasivayam, N. (2002). Hypolipidemic effect of Cuminum cyminum L. on alloxan-induced diabetic rats. *Pharmacol Res,* 46(3), 251-5.

357. Carlsen, M.H., Halvorsen, B.L., & Holte, K. (2010, July 22). The total antioxidant content of more than 3100 foods, beverages, spices, herbs and supplements used worldwide. *Nutr J,* 9, 3.

358. Bolkent, S., Yanardag, R., Ozsoy-Sacan, O., & Kara-bulut-Bulan, O. (2004). Effects of parsley (Petroselinum crispum) on the liver of diabetic rats: a morphological and biochemical study. *Phytother Res,* 18(12), 996-9.

359. Shukla, S., & Gupta, S. (2010). Apigenin: a promising molecule for cancer prevention. *Pharm Res,* 27(6):962-78.

360. World Health Organization (WHO). (2003). *Diet, nutrition and the prevention of chronic diseases: report of a joint WHO/FAO expert consultation.* Geneva: WHO.

361. World Health Organization (WHO). (2007). *Reducing Salt Intake in Populations: Report of a WHO Forum and Technical Meeting 5-7 October 2006, Paris, France.* Geneva: WHO.

362. Strazzullo, P., D'Elia, L., Kandala, N., & Cappuccio, F.P. (2009). Salt intake, stroke, and cardiovascular disease: meta-analysis of prospective studies. *Br Med J,* 339, b4567.

363. He, F.J., & MacGregor, G.A. (2007). Salt, blood pressure and cardiovascular disease. *Curr Opin Cardiol,* 22, 298-305.

364. De Wardener, H.E., & MacGregor, G.A. (2002). Harmful effects of dietary salt in addition to hypertension. *J Human Hypertension,* 16, 213-23.

365. Brown, I.J., Tzoulaki, I., Candeias, V., & Elliott, P. (2009). Salt intakes around the world: Implications for public health. *Int J Epidemiol,* 38, 791-813.

366. Woodruff, S.J., Fryer, K., & Campbell, T. (2014). Associations among blood pressure, salt consumption and body weight status of students from south-western Ontario. *Public Health Nutr,* 17(5), 1114–1119.

367. Graffe, C.C., Bech, J.N., & Pedersen, E.B. (2012). Effcet of high and low sodium intake on urinary aquaporin-2 excretion in healthy humans. *Am J Physiol,* 302(2), F264–F275.

368. Hulthén, L., Aurell, M., & Klingberg, S. (2010). Salt intake in young Swedish men. *Public Health Nutr,* 13(5), 601–605.

369. Prada, P., Okamoto, M.M., & Furukawa, L.N. (2000). High- or low-salt diet from weaning to adulthood: Effect on insulin sensitivity in wistar rats. *Hypertension,* 35(1 Pt 2), 424–429.

370. Coelho, M.S., Passadore, M.D., & Gasparetti, A.L. (2006). High- or low-salt diet from weaning to adulthood: Effect on body weight, food intake and energy balance in rats. *Nutr Metab Cardiovas,* 16(2), 148–155.

371. Zhao, D., Das, S., & Pandey, K.N. (2013). Interactive roles of Npr1 gene-dosage and salt diets on cardiac angiotensin II, aldosterone and pro-inflammatory cytokine levels in mutant null mice. *J Hypertens,* 31(1), 134–144.

372. Moritz, A. (2011, November 20). *The Benefits Of Sipping Hot, Ionized Water.* Retrieved from http://www.enerchi.com/the-benefits-of-sipping-hot-ionized-water/

373. Fukuchi, Y., Hiramitsu, M., & Okada, M. (2008). Lemon Polyphenols Suppress Diet-induced Obesity by Up-Regulation of mRNA Levels of the Enzymes Involved in beta-Oxidation in Mouse White Adipose Tissue. *J Clin Biochem Nutr*, 43(3), 201-9.

374. González-Molina, E., Domínguez-Perles, R., Moreno, D.A., & García-Viguera, C. (2010). Natural bioactive compounds of Citrus limon for food and health. *Journal of Pharmaceutical and Biomedical Analysis,* 51(2), 327–345.

375. Guyton, & Arthur, C. (1976). *Textbook of Medical Physiology (5th ed.).* Philadelphia: W.B. Saunders, 424.

376. Duff Conacher, Center for Study of Responsive Law. (1988). *The Nader report—Troubled waters on tap.* Washington (DC): Center for Study of Responsive Law.

377. Duff Conacher, Center for Study of Responsive Law. (1988). *Troubled waters on tap: Organic chemicals in public drinking ater systems and the failure of regulation.* Washington (DC): Center for Study of Responsive Law.

378. Duhigg, C. (2009, December 7). Millions in U.S. Drink Dirty Water, Records Show. *The New York Times.*

379. Rochester, J.R. (2013). Bisphenol A and human health: a review of the literature. *Reprod Toxicol,* 42, 132-55.

380. Ali, M. (2003). *Oxygen and aging.* New York: Canary 21 Press.

381. Wang, Z.Y., Zhou, Z.C., & Zhu, K.N. (2004). Microclustered water and hydration. *Asia Pac J Clin Nutr,* 13, S128.

382. Pan, J.G., Zhu, K.N., Zhou, M.C., & Wang, Z.Y. (2003). Low resonant frequency storage and transfer in structured water cluster. Systems, Man and Cybernetics. *IEEE International Conference on 2003.* 5, 5034–5039.

383. Katayama, S. (1992). Aging Mechanism Associated with a Function of Biowater. *Physiol Chem Phys Med NMR,* 24, 43–50.

384. Lee, K.J., Park, S.K., & Kim, J.W. (2004). Anticancer effect of alkaline reduced water. *J Int Soc Life Inf Sci,* 22, 302–305.

385. Jin, D., Ryu, S.H., & Kim, H.W. (2006). Anti-diabetic effect of alkaline-reduced water on OLETF rats. *Biosci Biotechonol Biochem,* 70, 31–37.

386. Li, Y., Hamasaki, T., & Nakamichi, N. (2011). Suppressive effects of electrolyzed reduced water on alloxan-induced apoptosis and type 1 diabetes mellitus. *Cytotechnology,* 63, 119–131.

387. Ye, J., Li, Y., & Hamasaki, T. (2008). Inhibitory effect of electrolyzed reduced water on tumor angiogenesis. *Biol Pharmaceut Bull,* 31, 19–26.

388. Boschmann, M., Steiniger, J., & Hille, U. (2003). Water-induced thermogenesis. *J Clin Endocrinol Metab,* 88(12), 6015-9.

389. Davy, B.M., Dennis, E.A., Dengo, A.L., Wilson, K.L., & Davy, K.P. (2008). Water consumption reduces energy intake at a breakfast meal in obese older adults. *J Am Diet Assoc,* 108(7), 1236-9.

390. Dennis, E.A., Dengo, A.L., & Comber, D.L. (2010). Water consumption increases weight loss during a hypocaloric diet intervention in middle-aged and older adults. *Obesity (Silver Spring),* 18(2), 300-7.

CHAPTER 3: LIFESTYLE

1. Thorogood, A., Mottillo, S., & Shimony, A. (2011). Isolated aerobic exercise and weight loss: a systematic review and meta-analysis of randomized controlled trials. *Am J Med,* 124(8), 747-55.

2. Van Reeth, O., Sturis, J., & Byrne, M.M. (1994). Nocturnal exercise phase delays circadian rhythms of melatonin and thyrotropin secretion in normal men. *Am J Physiol,* 266(6 Pt 1), E964-74.

3. Kushi, L. H. (1997). Physical activity and mortality in postmenopausal women. *Journal of the American Medical Association,* 277(16), 1287–92.

4. Sherman, S. E., D'Agostino, R. B., Cobb, J. L., & Kannel, W. B. (1994). Physical activity and mortality in women in the Framingham Heart Study. *American Heart Journal,* 128(5), 879–84.

5. Blair, S. N., Kohl, H. W III, Barlow, C. E., Paffenbarger Jr., R. S., Gibbons L. W., & Macera, C. A. (1995). Changes in physical fitness and all-cause mortality. A prospective study of healthy and unhealthy men. *Journal of the American Medical Association,* 273(14), 1093–98.

6. Warburton, D. E., Nicol, C. W., & Bredin, S. S. (2006). Health benefits of physical activity: The evidence. *Canadian Medical Association Journal,* 174(6), 801–9.

7. Radak, Z., Chung, H. Y., & Goto, S. (2005). Exercise and hormesis: Oxidative stress-related adaptation for successful aging. *Biogerontology,* 6(1), 71–75.

8. Castillo-Garzón, M. J., Ruiz, J. R., Ortega, F. B., & Gutiérrez, Á. (2006). Anti-aging therapy through fitness enhancement. *Journal of Clinical Interventions in Aging,* 1(3), 213–20.

9. Puterman, E., Lin, J., Blackburn, E., O'Donovan, A., Adler, N., & Epel, E. (2010). The power of exercise: buffering the effect of chronic stress on telomere length. *PLoS One,* 5(5), e10837.

10. Donnelly, J.E., Hill, J.O., & Jacobsen, D.J. (2003). Effects of a 16-month randomized controlled exercise trial on body weight and composition in young, overweight men and women: the Midwest Exercise Trial. *Arch Intern Med,* 163(11), 1343-1350.

11. McGuire, M.T., Wing, R.R., Klem, M.L., Seagle, H.M., & Hill, J.O. (1998). Long-term maintenance of weight loss: Do people who lose weight through various weight loss methods use different behaviors to maintain their weight? *Int J Obes Relat Metab Disord,* 22(6), 572-7.

12. O'Keefe, J.H., Patil, H.R., Lavie, C.J., Magalski, A., Vogel, R.A., & McCullough, P.A. (2012). Potential adverse cardiovascular effects from excessive endurance exercise. *Mayo Clin Proc,* 87, 587–95.

13. Schnohr, P., O'Keefe, J.H., Marott, J.L., Lange, P., & Jensen, G.B. (2015). Dose of jogging and long-term mortality: the Copenhagen City Heart Study. *J Am Coll Cardiol,* 65(5), 411-9.

14. Shave, R., Baggish, A., George, K. (2010). Exercise-induced cardiac troponin elevation: evidence, mechanisms, and implications. *J Am Coll Cardiol,* 56, 169–76.

15. Shaw, K., Gennet, H., O'Rourke, P., Del Mar, C. (2006). Exercise for Overweight or Obesity. *The Cochrane Collaboration,* 18(4), CD003817.

16. Wu, T., Gao, X., Chen, M., Van Dam, R.M. (2009). Long-term effectiveness of diet-plus-exercise interventions

vs. diet-only interventions for weight loss: a meta-analysis: obesity Management. *Obesity Reviews,* 10(3), 313–323.

17. Moritz, A. (2005). *Timeless Secrets of Health and Rejuvenation.* Ener-chi.

18. Boutcher, S.H. (2011). High-intensity intermittent exercise and fat loss. *J Obes,* 868305.

19. Shaw, K., Gennat, H., O'Rourke, P., Del Mar, C. (2006). Exercise for overweight or obesity. *Cochrane Database Syst Rev,* (4), CD003817.

20. Roberts, L.D., Boström, P., & O'Sullivan, J.F. (2014). β-Aminoisobutyric acid induces browning of white fat and hepatic β-oxidation and is inversely correlated with cardiometabolic risk factors. *Cell Metab,* 19(1), 96-108.

21. Sevits, K.J., Melanson, E.L., & Swibas, T. (2013). Total daily energy expenditure is increased following a single bout of sprint interval training. *Physiol Rep,* 1(5), e00131.

22. Gibala, M.J., & McGee, S.L. (2008). Metabolic adaptations to short-term high-intensity interval training: a little pain for a lot of gain? *Exercise and Sport Sciences Review,* 36(2), 58–63.

23. Trapp, E.G., Chisholm, D.J., Freund, J., & Boutcher, S.H. (2008). The effects of high-intensity intermittent exercise training on fat loss and fasting insulin levels of young women. *International Journal of Obesity,* 32(4), 684–691.

24. Bryant, J. (2015, March 27). *11 Fat Loss Rules: What To Consider While Keeping Muscle!* Retrieved from http://www.bodybuilding.com/fun/11_fat_loss_rules.htm

25. Gonzalez, J. T. (2013). Breakfast and exercise contingently affect postprandial metabolism and energy balance in physically active males. *Br J Nutr,* 23, 1-12.

26. Stoppani, Jim. (2015, March 18). *Is Fasted Cardio The Best For Burning Fat?* Retrieved from http://www.bodybuilding.com/fun/is-fasted-cardio-the-best-for-burning-fat.html

27. Wang, Z., Ying, Z., & Bosy-westphal, A. (2011). Evaluation of specific metabolic rates of major organs and tissues: comparison between men and women. *Am J Hum Biol*, 23(3), 333-8.

28. Patrick, R. (2015, March 19). *6 Compound Training Movements Build Serious Mass!* Retrieved from http://www.bodybuilding.com/fun/6-compound-movements-build-mass.htm

29. *Movement Patterns: Exercises For Horizontal & Vertical Push & Pull, Quad & Hip Dominant, And More.* Retrieved from http://www.aworkoutroutine.com/movement-patterns/

30. Klem, M.L., Wing, R.R., McGuire, M.T., Seagle, H.M., & Hill, J.O. (1997). A descriptive study of individuals successful at long-term maintenance of substantial weight loss. *American Journal of Clinical Nutrition, 66*, 239-246.

31. Shick, S.M., Wing, R.R., Klem, M.L., McGuire, M.T., Hill, J.O., & Seagle, H.M. (1998). Persons successful at long-term weight loss and maintenance continue to consume a low calorie, low fat diet. *Journal of the American Dietetic Association, 98*, 408-413.

32. Plante, T.G., Gustafson, C., Brecht, C., Imberi, J., & Sanchez, J. (2011). Exercising with an iPod, friend, or neither: which is better for psychological benefits? *Am J Health Behav*, 35(2), 199-208.

33. *Exercise and Depression.* Retrieved from http://www.webmd.com/depression/guide/exercise-depression

34. Carter, A. E. (1979). *The Miracles of Rebound Exercise.* Washington: The National institute of Reboundology and Health, Inc.

35. McGlone, C., L. Kravitz, J. J., & Janot J. (2002). Rebounding exercise versus treadmill jogging: A cardiorespiratory comparison. *Medicine and Science In Sports and Exercise,* 34(5).

36. McGlone, C., Kravitz, L., & Janot, J. (2002). Rebounding: A low-impact exercise alternative. *ACSM's Health & Fitness Journal,* 6(2), 11–15.

37. Richardson, S. D. (2010). What's in the pool? A comprehensive identification of disinfection by-products and assessment of mutagenicity of chlorinated and brominated swimming pool water. *Environmental Health Perspectives,* 118(11), 1523–30.

38. Zwiener, C., Richardson, S. D., DeMarini, D. M, Grummt, T., Glauner, T., & Frimmel, F. H. (2007). Drowning in disinfection byproducts? Assessing swimming pool water. *Environmental Science and Technology,* 41(2), 363–72.

39. Raloff, J. (1986). Toxic showers And baths, *Science News,* 130, 190.

40. Anderson, I. (1986). Showers Pose a Risk to Health. *New Scientist,* 18.

41. Larkey, L., Jahnke, R., Etnier, J., & Gonzalez, J. (2009). Meditative movement as a category of exercise: Implications for research. *Journal of Physical Activity and Health,* 6(2), 230–38.

42. Hefen, X., Huining, X., Meiguang, B., Chengming, Z., & Shuying, Z. (1993). Clinical study of the anti-aging effect of

qigong. *Proceedings, Second World Conference for Academic Exchange of Medical Qigong.* Beijing, China, 137.

43. Kuang, A., Wang, C., Xu, D., & Qian, Y. (1991). Research on the anti-aging effect of qigong. *Journal of Traditional Chinese Medicine,* 11(2), 153–58.

44. Sancier, K. M., & Holman, D. (2004). Multifaceted health benefits of medical qigong. *Journal of Alternative and Complementary Medicine,* 10(1), 163–65.

45. Jahnke, R., Larkey, L., Rogers, C., Etnier, J., & Lin, F. (2010). A comprehensive review of health benefits of qigong and tai chi. *American Journal of Health Promotion,* 24(6), e1–e25.

46. Ross, A., & Thomas, S. (2010). The health benefits of yoga and exercise: a review of comparison studies. *Journal of Alternative and Complementary Medicine,* 16(1), 3–12.

47. Woodyard, C. (2011). Exploring the therapeutic effects of yoga and its ability to increase quality of life. *International Journal of Yoga,* 4(2), 49–54.

48. Manchanda, S. C. (2000). Retardation of coronary atherosclerosis with yoga lifestyle intervention. *Journal of Association of Physicians of India,* 48(7), 687–94.

49. Michalsen, A. (2005). Rapid stress reduction and anxiolysis among distressed women as a consequence of a three-month intensive yoga program. *Medical Science Monitor,* 11(12), CR555–61.

50. Saat, M., Singh, R., Sirisinghe, R.G., & Nawawi, M. (2002). Rehydration after exercise with fresh young coconut water, carbohydrate-electrolyte beverage and plain water. *J Physiol Anthropol Appl Human Sci,* 21(2), 93-104.

51. McGuire, M.T., Wing, R.R., Klem, M.L., & Hill, J.O. (1999). Behavioral strategies of individuals who have maintained long-term weight losses. *Obes Res,* 7(4), 334-41.

52. Linde, J.A., Jeffery, R.W., French, S.A., Pronk, N.P., & Boyle, R.G. (2005). Self-weighing in weight gain prevention and weight loss trials. *Ann Behav Med,* 30, 210–216.

53. Butryn, M.L., Phelan, S., Hill, J.O., & Wing, R.R. (2007). Consistent self-monitoring of weight: a key component of successful weight loss maintenance. *Obesity (Silver Spring),* 15, 3091 -3096.

54. Linde, J.A., Jeffery, R.W., & Finch, E,A. (2007). Relation of body mass index to depression and weighing frequency in overweight women. *Prev Med,* 45(1), 75-9.

55. Regan, J. *One pound of fat versus one pound of muscle clearing up the misconception.* Retrieved from http://bamboocorefitness.com/one-pound-of-fat-versus-one-pound-of-muscle-clearing-up-the-misconception/

56. Kamb, S. (2012, July 2) *Everything You Need to Know About Body Fat Percentage.* Retrieved from http://www.nerdfitness.com/blog/2012/07/02/body-fat-percentage/

57. Frisch, R.E. (1987). Body fat, menarche, fitness and fertility. *Hum Reprod,* 2(6), 521-33.

58. *Percent Body Fat Calculator: Skinfold Method.* Retrieved from http://www.acefitness.org/acefit/healthy_living_tools_content.aspx?id=2

59. Andersen, C. (2012, June 1). *The Best (and Worst) Ways to Measure Body Fat.* Retrieved from http://www.shape.com/weight-loss/weight-loss-strategies/best-and-worst-ways-measure-body-fat

60. Centers for Disease Control, Prevention. (2011, March 4). *Effect of short sleep duration on daily activities–United States.* MMWR Morb Mortal Wkly Rep, 60, 239–242.

61. Chao, C.Y., Wu, J.S., & Yang, Y.C. (2011). Sleep duration is a potential risk factor for newly diagnosed type 2 diabetes mellitus. *Metabolism,* 60, 799–804.

62. Wang, Q., Xi, B., Liu, M., Zhang, Y., & Fu, M. (2012). Short sleep duration is associated with hypertension risk among adults: a systematic review and meta-analysis. *Hypertens Res,* 35, 1012–1018.

63. Cappuccio, F.P., D'Elia, L., Strazzullo, P., & Miller, M.A. (2010). Sleep duration and all-cause mortality: a systematic review and meta-analysis of prospective studies. *Sleep,* 33, 585–592.

64. Patel, S.R., Hu, F.B. (2008). Short sleep duration and weight gain: a systematic review. *Obesity (Silver Spring),* 16, 643-53.

65. Pan, A., Schernhammer, E.S., Sun, Q., & Hu, F.B. (2011). Rotating night shift work and risk of type 2 diabetes: two prospective cohort studies in women. *PLoS Med,* 8, e1001141.

66. Costa, G., Haus, E., & Stevens, R. (2010). Shift work and cancer—considerations on rationale, mechanisms, and epidemiology. *Scand J Work Environ Health,* 36, 163–179.

67. Straif, K., Baan, R., & Grosse, Y. (2007). Carcinogenicity of shift-work, painting, and firefighting. *Lancet Oncol,* 8, 1065–1066.

68. Spaeth, A.M., Dinges, D.F., & Goel, N. (2013). Effects of Experimental Sleep Restriction on Weight Gain, Caloric Intake, and Meal Timing in Healthy Adults. *Sleep,* 36(7), 981-990.

69. Kobayashi, D., Takahashi, O., Deshpande, G.A., Shimbo, T., & Fukui, T. (2012). Association between weight gain, obesity, and sleep duration: a large-scale 3-year cohort study. *Sleep Breath,* 16, 829–833.

70. Patel, S.R., Malhotra, A., White, D.P., Gottlieb, D.J., & Hu, F.B. (2006). Association between reduced sleep and weight gain in women. *Am J Epidemiol,* 164, 947-54.

71. Kooijman, S., Van den Berg, R., & Ramkisoensing, A. (2015). Prolonged daily light exposure increases body fat mass through attenuation of brown adipose tissue activity. *Proc Natl Acad Sci U S A,* 112(21), 6748-53.

72. Borniger, J.C., Maurya, S.K., Periasamy, M., & Nelson, R.J. (2014). Acute dim light at night increases body mass, alters metabolism, and shifts core body temperature circadian rhythms. *Chronobiol Int,* 31(8), 917-25.

73. Goel, N., Kim, H., & Lao, R.P. (2005). An olfactory stimulus modifies nighttime sleep in young men and women. *Chronobiol Int,* 22(5), 889-904.

74. *How Much Sleep Do We Really Need?* Retrieved from http://sleepfoundation.org/how-sleep-works/how-much-sleep-do-we-really-need

75. Biddle, J.E., Hamermesh, D.S. (1990). Sleep and the allocation of time. *J Polit Econ,* 98, 922–943.

76. Basner, M., Fomberstein, K.M., & Razavi, F.M. (2007). American time use survey: sleep time and its relationship to waking activities. *Sleep,* 30, 1085–1095.

77. Huang, H.W., Zheng, B.L., & Jiang, L. (2015). Effect of oral melatonin and wearing earplugs and eye masks on nocturnal sleep in healthy subjects in a simulated intensive care unit environment: which might be a more promising strategy for ICU sleep deprivation? *Crit Care,* 19, 124.

78. Hu, R.F., Jiang, X.Y., Zeng, Y.M., Chen, X.Y., & Zhang, Y.H. (2010). Effects of earplugs and eye masks on nocturnal sleep, melatonin and cortisol in a simulated intensive care unit environment. *Crit Care,* 14, R66.

CHAPTER 4: SUPPLEMENTS

1. Liu, R. H. (2004). Potential synergy of phytochemicals in cancer prevention: Mechanism of action. *The Journal of Nutrition,* 134(12), 3479S–3485S.

2. Thiel, R. J. (2000). Natural vitamins may be superior to synthetic ones. *Medical Hypotheses,* 55(6), 461–69.

3. King, J. C, Cousins, R. J., Olsen, J.A., Shike, M., & Ross, A.C. (2005*). Modern Nutrition in Health and Disease,* (10) 271–85. Philadelphia: Lipponcott, Williams and Wilkins.

4. Astrup, A., Toubro, S., Christensen, N.J., & Quaade, F. (1992). Pharmacology of thermogenic drugs. *Am J Clin Nutr,* 55(1 Suppl), 246S-248S.

5. Astrup, A., Toubro, S., Cannon, S., Hein, P., Breum, L., & Madsen, J. (1990). Caffeine: a double-blind, placebo-controlled study of its thermogenic, metabolic, and cardiovascular effects in healthy volunteers. *Am J Clin Nutr,* 51(5), 759-67.

6. Between basal metabolic rate, thermogenic response to caffeine, and body weight loss following combined low calorie and exercise treatment in obese women. (1994). *Int J Obes Relat Metab Disord,* 18(5), 345-50.

7. Dulloo, A.G., Geissler, C.A., Horton, T., Collins, A., & Miller, D.S. (1989). Normal caffeine consumption: influence on thermogenesis and daily energy expenditure in lean and postobese human volunteers. *Am J Clin Nutr,* 49(1), 44-50.

8. Preuss, H.G., DiFerdinando, D., Bagchi, M., & Bagchi, D. (2002). Citrus aurantium as a thermogenic, weight-reduction

replacement for ephedra: an overview. *J Med,* 33(1-4), 247-64.

9. Stohs, S.J., Preuss, H.G., & Shara, M. (2012, August 29). A review of the human clinical studies involving Citrus aurantium (bitter orange) extract and its primary protoalkaloid p-synephrine. *Int J Med Sci,* 9(7), 527-38.

10. Saper, R.B., Eisenberg, D.M., & Phillips, R.S. (2004, November 1). Common dietary supplements for weight loss. *Am Fam Physician,* 70(9), 1731-8.

11. Nachtigal, M.C., Patterson, R.E., Stratton, K.L., Adams, L.A., & Shattuck, A.L. (2005). White E. Dietary supplements and weight control in a middle-age population. *J Altern Complement Med,* 11(5):909-15.

12. Anderson, R.A. (1998). Effects of chromium on body composition and weight loss. *Nutr Rev,* 56(9), 266-70.

13. Song, M.Y., Kim, B.S., & Kim, H. (2014). Influence of Panax ginseng on obesity and gut microbiota in obese middle-aged Korean women. *J Ginseng Res,* 38(2), 106-15.

14. Hursel, R., Viechtbauer, W., & Westerterp-Plantenga, M.S. (2009). The effects of green tea on weight loss and weight maintenance: a meta-analysis. *Int J Obes (Lond),* 33(9), 956-61.

15. Onakpoya, I., Hung, S.K., Perry, R., Wider, B., & Ernst, E. (2011). The Use of Garcinia Extract (Hydroxycitric Acid) as a Weight loss Supplement: A Systematic Review and Meta-Analysis of Randomised Clinical Trials. *J Obes,* 509038.

16. Frati-Munari, A.C., Fernández-Harp, J.A., Becerril, M., Chávez-Negrete, A., Bañales-Ham, M. (1983). Decrease in serum lipids, glycemia and body weight by Plantago psyllium in obese and diabetic patients. *Arch Invest Med (Mex),* 14(3), 259-68.

17. Onakpoya, I., Terry, R., & Ernst, E. (2011). The use of green coffee extract as a weight loss supplement: a systematic review and meta-analysis of randomised clinical trials. *Gastroenterol Res Pract,* 382852.

18. Cowan, T. (2004). *The Fourfold Path to Healing: Working with the Laws of Nutrition, Therapeutics, Movement and Meditation in the Art of Medicine.* Newtrends Publishing.

19. Morimoto, C., Satoh, Y., & Hara, M. (2005, May 27). Anti-obese action of raspberry ketone. *Life Sci,* 77(2), 194-204.

20. Park, K.S. (2010). Raspberry ketone increases both lipolysis and fatty acid oxidation in 3T3-L1 adipocytes. *Planta Med,* 76(15), 1654-8.

21. Lopez, H.L., Ziegenfuss, T.N., & Hofheins, J.E. (2013). Eight weeks of supplementation with a multi-ingredient weight loss product enhances body composition, reduces hip and waist girth, and increases energy levels in overweight men and women. *J Int Soc Sports Nutr,* 10(1), 22.

22. Slavin, J.L. (2005). Dietary fiber and body weight. *Nutrition,* 21(3), 411-8.

23. Anderson, J. W., Baird, P., Davis, R. H. Jr, Ferreri, S., Knudtson, M., Koraym, A., ...Williams, C. L. (2009). Health benefits of dietary fiber. *Nutrition Reviews,* 67(4), 188-205.

24. Heber, D. (2003). Herbal preparations for obesity: are they useful? *Prim Care,* 30(2), 441-63.

25. Van Heerden, F.R. (2008, October 28). Hoodia gordonii: a natural appetite suppressant. *J Ethnopharmacol,* 119(3), 434-7.

26. Van Heerden, F.R., Marthinus, H.R., & Maharaj, V.J. (2007). An appetite suppressant from Hoodia species. *Phytochemistry,* 68(20), 2545-53.

27. Lee, R.A., & Balick, M.J. (2007). Indigenous use of Hoodia gordonii and appetite suppression. *Explore (NY),* 3(4), 404-6.

28. Haskell, C. F., Kennedy, D. O., Wesnes, K. A., Milne, A. L., & Scholey, A. B. (2007). A double-blind, placebo-controlled, multi-dose evaluation of the acute behavioural effects of guaraná in humans. *Journal of Psychopharmacology,* 21(1), 65–70.

29. Enkovaara, A.L. (2010). With red rice against cholesterol? *Duodecim,* 126(6), 623-6.

30. de Leiris, J., de Lorgeril, M., & Boucher, F. (2009). Fish oil and heart health. *J Cardiovasc Pharmacol,* 54(5), 378-384.

31. Brinson, B.E., & Miller, S. (2012). Fish oil: what is the role in cardiovascular health? *J Pharm Pract,* 25(1), 69-74.

32. Montori, V.M., Farmer, A., Wollan, P.C., & Dinneen, S.F. (2000). Fish oil supplementation in type 2 diabetes: a quantitative systematic review. *Diabetes Care,* 23(9), 1407-15.

33. Patel, D.K., Prasad, S.K., Kumar, R., & Hemalatha, S. (2012). An overview on antidiabetic medicinal plants having insulin mimetic property. *Asian Pac J Trop Biomed,* 2(4), 320-30.

34. Kumar, V., Bhandari, U., Tripathi, C.D., & Khanna, G. (2013). Anti-obesity Effect of Gymnema sylvestre Extract on High Fat Diet-induced Obesity in Wistar Rats. *Drug Res (Stuttg),* 63(12), 625-32.

35. Leach, M.J. (2007). Gymnema sylvestre for diabetes mellitus: a systematic review. *J Altern Complement Med,* 13(9), 977-83.

36. *Gymnema (Gymnema sylvestre).* Retrieved from http://restorativemedicine.org/books/healing-diabetes-complementary-naturopathic-and-drug-treatments/botanical-medicine-therapy/gymnema-gymnema-sylvestre/

37. Liu, R. H. (2003). Health benefits of fruit and vegetables are from additive and synergistic combinations of phytochemicals. *The American Society for Clinical Nutrition,* 78(3), 517S-520S.

38. Liu, R. H. (2004). Potential synergy of phytochemicals in cancer prevention: mechanism of action. *The Journal of Nutrition,* 134(12), 3479S-3485S.

39. Baile, C.A., Yang, J.Y., Rayalam, S., Hartzell, D.L., Lai, C.Y., Andersen, C., & Della-Fera, M.A. (2011). Effect of resveratrol on fat mobilization. *Ann N Y Acad Sci,* 1215, 40-7.

40. Timmers, S., Konings, E., & Bilet, L. (2011). Calorie restriction-like effects of 30 days of resveratrol supplementation on energy metabolism and metabolic profile in obese humans. *Cell Metab,* 14(5), 612-22.

41. Bradford, P. G. (2013). Curcumin and obesity. *Biofactors,* 39(1), 78-87.

42. Zhang, D.W., Fu, M., Gao, S.H., & Liu, J.L. (2013). Curcumin and diabetes: a systematic review. *Evid Based Complement Alternat Med,* 636053.

43. Wongcharoen, W., Phrommintikul, A. (2009, April 3). The protective role of curcumin in cardiovascular diseases. *Int J Cardiol,* 133(2), 145-51.

44. Srivastava, J.K., Shankar, E., Gupta, S. (2010, November 1). Chamomile: A herbal medicine of the past with bright future. *Mol Med Rep,* 3(6), 895-901.

45. Gershwin, M. E., & Amha Belay. (2008). *Spirulina in human nutrition and health.* Boca Raton: CRC Press.

46. Ciferri, O. (1983). Spirulina, the edible microorganism. *Microbiological Reviews,* 47(4), 551–78.

47. Babadzhanov, A. S., Abdusamatova, N., Yusupova, F. M., Faizullaeva, N., Mezhlumyan, L. G., & Malikova, M. K. (2004). Chemical composition of Spirulina platensis cultivated in Uzbekistan. *Chemistry of Natural Compounds,* 40(3), 276–79.

48. Belay, A. (2002). The potential application of Spirulina (Arthrospira) as a nutritional and therapeutic supplement in health management. *Journal of the American Nutraceutical Association,* 5(2), 27-48.

49. Goodhart, S. R., & Shils, E. M. (1980). *Modern nutrition in health and disease. (6th ed.).* Philadelphia: Lea and Febinger, 134–38.

50. Simopoulos, A. P. (2002). Omega-3 fatty acids in inflammation and autoimmune diseases. *Journal of the American College of Nutrition,* 21(6), 495-505.

51. Francois, C. A., Connor, S. L., Bolewicz, L. C., & Connor, W. E. (2003). Supplementing lactating women with flaxseed oil does not increase docosahexaenoic acid in their milk. *American Journal of Clinical Nutrition,* 77(1), 226–33.

52. Khani, S., Hosseini, H. M., Taheri, M., Nourani, M. R., & Imani Fooladi, A. A. (2012). Probiotics as an alternative strategy for prevention and treatment of human diseases: A review. *Inflammation and Allergy Drug Targets,* 11(2), 79–89.

53. Yan, F., & Polk, D. B. (2011). Probiotics and immune health. *Current Opinion In Gastroenterology,* 27(6), 496–501.

54. Douillard, J. (2014, September 4). *How to Choose the Right Probiotic for Your Imbalance.* Retrieved from http://lifespa.com/choose-right-probiotic-imbalance/

CHAPTER 5: HIDDEN FACTORS

1. Cuthbert, S. C., & Goodheart, G. J. Jr. (2007). On the reliability and validity of manual muscle testing: A literature review. *Chiropractic and Osteopathy,* 15(4).

2. Després, J.P. (2007). Cardiovascular disease under the influence of excess visceral fat. *Crit Pathw Cardiol,* 6(2), 51-9.

3. Gholap, S., & Kar, A. (2004). Hypoglycaemic effects of some plant extracts are possibly mediated through inhibition in corticosteroid concentration. *Pharmazie,* 59, 876–8.

4. Cohen, M.M. (2014). Tulsi - Ocimum sanctum: A herb for all reasons. *J Ayurveda Integr Med,* 5(4), 251-9.

5. Cohen, G., Shamus, E. (2009). Depressed, Low Self-Esteem: What can exercise do for you? *The Internet Journal of Allied Health Sciences and Practice,* 7(2).

6. Hill, E.E., Zack, E., Battaglini, C., Viru, M., Viru, A., & Hackney, A.C. (2008). Exercise and circulating cortisol levels: the intensity threshold effect. *J Endocrinol Invest,* 31(7), 587-91.

7. Leproult, R., Copinschi, G., Buxton, O., & Van Cauter, E. (1997). Sleep loss results in an elevation of cortisol levels the next evening. *Sleep,* 20(10), 865-70.

8. Seelig, M.S. (1994). Consequences of magnesium deficiency on the enhancement of stress reactions; preventive

and therapeutic implications (a review). *J Am Coll Nutr,* 13(5), 429-46.

9. Dean, C. (2006). *The Magnesium Miracle.* Ballantine Books.

10. Humphries, S., Kushner, H., & Falkner, B. (1999). Low dietary magnesium is associated with insulin resistance in a sample of young, nondiabetic Black Americans. *Am J Hypertens,* 12(8 Pt 1), 747-56.

11. LeBlanc, E.S., Rizzo, J.H., & Pedula, K.L. (2012). Associations between 25-hydroxyvitamin D and weight gain in elderly women. *J Women's Health (Larchmt),* 21(10), 1066-73.

12. Murray, M., & Pizzorno, J. (1998). *Encyclopedia of Natural Medicine* (2nd ed.). New York: Three Rivers Press.

13. Kalsbeek, A., la Fleur, S., & Fliers, E. (2014, March 19). Circadian control of glucose metabolism. *Mol Metab,* 3(4), 372-83.

14. Mehran, A.E., Templeman, N.M., & Brigidi, G.S. (2012, December 5). Hyperinsulinemia drives diet-induced obesity independently of brain insulin production. *Cell Metab,* 16(6), 723-37.

15. Shanmugasundaram, E.R., Gopinath, K.L., Radha Shanmugasundaram, K., & Rajendran, V.M. (1990). Possible regeneration of the islets of Langerhans in streptozotocin-diabetic rats given Gymnema sylvestre leaf extracts. *J Ethnopharmacol,* 30(3), 265-79.

16. Sullivan, P.B. (1999). Food allergy and food intolerance in childhood. *Indian J Pediatr,* 66(1), S37-45.

17. Gotua, M., Lomidze, N., Dolidze, N., & Gotua, T. (2008). IgE-mediated food hypersensitivity disorders. *Georgian Med News*, (157), 39-44.

18. Speer, F. (1976). Food allergy: the 10 common offenders. *Am Fam Physician*, 13(2), 106-12.

19. Ito, K. (2015). Grain and legume allergy. *Chem Immunol Allergy*, 101, 145-51.

20. Colin, P. (2006). Homeopathy and respiratory allergies: A series of 147 cases. *Homeopathy*, 95(2), 68–72.

21. Riley, D., Fischer, M., Singh, B., Haidvogl, M., & Heger, M. (2001). Homeopathy and conventional medicine: An outcomes study comparing effectiveness in a primary care setting. *Journal of Alternative and Complementary Medicine*, 7(2), 149–59.

22. Baillie-Hamilton, P.F. (2002). Chemical toxins: a hypothesis to explain the global obesity epidemic. *J Altern Complement Med*, 8(2), 185-92.

23. Fukuchi, Y., Hiramitsu, M., & Okada, M. (2008). Lemon Polyphenols Suppress Diet-induced Obesity by Up-Regulation of mRNA Levels of the Enzymes Involved in beta-Oxidation in Mouse White Adipose Tissue. *J Clin Biochem Nutr*, 43(3), 201-9.

24. Kim, M.J., Hwang, J.H., & Ko, H.J. (2015). Lemon detox diet reduced body fat, insulin resistance, and serum hs-CRP level without hematological changes in overweight Korean women. *Nutr Res*, 35(5), 409-20.

25. Conterno, L., Fava, F., Viola, R., & Tuohy, K.M. (2011). Obesity and the gut microbiota: does up-regulating colonic fermentation protect against obesity and metabolic disease? *Genes Nutr*, 6(3), 241-60.

26. Schilder, R.J., Marden, J.H. (2006). Metabolic syndrome and obesity in an insect. *Proc Natl Acad Sci U S A,* 103(49), 18805-9.

27. Pearce, E.N. (2012). Thyroid hormone and obesity. *Curr Opin Endocrinol Diabetes Obes,* 19(5), 408-13.

28. Terrón, M.P., Delgado-Adámez, J., & Pariente, J.A. (2013, July 13). Melatonin reduces body weight gain and increases nocturnal activity in male Wistar rats. *Physiol Behav,* 118, 8-13.

29. Ceci, F., Cangiano, C., & Cairella, M. (1989). The effects of oral 5-hydroxytryptophan administration on feeding behavior in obese adult female subjects. *J Neural Transm,* 76(2), 109-17.

30. Wurtman, J.J. (1993). Depression and weight gain: the serotonin connection. *J Affect Disord,* 29(2-3), 183-92.

31. Traish, A.M. (2014). Testosterone and weight loss: the evidence. *Curr Opin Endocrinol Diabetes Obes,* 21(5), 313-22.

32. Chandeying, V., Sangthawan, M. (2007). Efficacy comparison of Pueraria mirifica (PM) against conjugated equine estrogen (CEE) with/without medroxyprogesterone acetate (MPA) in the treatment of climacteric symptoms in perimenopausal women: phase III study. *Journal of the Medical Association of Thailand,* 90(9), 1720–26.

33. Klok, M.D., Jakobsdottir, S., & Drent, M.L. (2007). The role of leptin and ghrelin in the regulation of food intake and body weight in humans: a review. *Obes Rev,* 8(1), 21-34.

34. Jung, C.H., & Kim, M.S. (2013). Molecular mechanisms of central leptin resistance in obesity. *Arch Pharm Res,* 36(2), 201-7.

35. Taheri, S., Lin, L., Austin, D., Young, T., & Mignot, E. (2004). Short sleep duration is associated with reduced leptin, elevated ghrelin, and increased body mass index. *PLoS Med,* 1(3), e62.

36. Kruse, J. (2011, June 29). *My Leptin Prescription.* Retrieved from https://www.jackkruse.com/my-leptin-prescription

37. Felitti, V.J. (1991). Long-term medical consequences of incest, rape, and molestation. *South Med J,* 84(3), 328–31.

38. Matthews, K.A., Räikkönen, K., Gallo, L., & Kuller, L.H. (2008). Association between socioeconomic status and metabolic syndrome in women: testing the reserve capacity model. *Health Psychol,* 27(5), 576-83.

39. Oliver, G., Wardle, J., & Gibson, E.L. (2000). Stress and food choice: a laboratory study. *Psychosom Med,* 62(6), 853-65.

40. Timmerman, G.M., & Acton, G.J. (2001). The relationship between basic need satisfaction and emotional eating. *Issues Ment Health Nurs,* 22(7), 691-701.

41. Felitti, V.J., Jakstis, K., Pepper, V., & Ray, A. (2010). Obesity: problem, solution, or both? *Perm J,* 14(1), 24-30.

42. Smith, A. (2010, July 25). *Experts see strong link between sexual abuse and obesity.* Retrieved from http://www.syracuse.com/news/index.ssf/2010/07/linking_sexual_abuse_to_obesit.html

43. Grossman, P., Niemann, L., Schmidt, S., & Walach, H. (2004). Mindfulness-based stress reduction and health benefits. A meta-analysis. *J Psychosom Res,* 57(1), 35-43.

44. Olson, K.L., & Emery, C.F. (2015). Mindfulness and weight loss: a systematic review. *Psychosom Med,* 77(1), 59-67.

45. Camilleri, G.M., Méjean, C., Bellisle, F., Hercberg, S., & Péneau, S. (2015). Association between Mindfulness and Weight Status in a General Population from the NutriNet-Santé Study. *PLoS One,* 10(6), e0127447.

46. Daubenmier, J., Kristeller, J., & Hecht, F.M. (2011). Mindfulness Intervention for Stress Eating to Reduce Cortisol and Abdominal Fat among Overweight and Obese Women: An Exploratory Randomized Controlled Study. *J Obes,* 651936.

47. Loyd, A. (2013). *The Healing Code: 6 Minutes to Heal the Source of Your Health, Success, or Relationship Issue.* Grand Central Life & Style.

48. Stahre, L. (2005). A short-term cognitive group treatment program gives substantial weight reduction up to 18 months from the end of treatment. A randomized controlled trial. *Eating and Weight Disorders,* 10, 51-58.

49. Wurtman, R.J. (1986). Ways that foods can affect the brain. *Nutr Rev,* 44, 2-6.